Saving Legs,

Saving Lives . . .

Peripheral Vascular Disease Made Simple

Saving Legs, Saving Lives:
Peripheral Vascular Disease Made Simple
First Edition

Midwest Cardiovascular
Research Foundation

Copyright © 2010
Midwest Cardiovascular Research Foundation
1622 E Lombard Street
Davenport, Iowa 52803
Phone: 563-324-2828
Fax: 563-324-2835
www.mcrfmd.com

ISBN 978-0-9755384-3-2

The reader is urged to review the package information data of the
manufacturers of any products mentioned.

Printed in the United States of America

Midwest Cardiovascular Research Foundation
1622 E Lombard Street
Davenport, Iowa 52803
Phone: 563-324-2828
Fax: 563-324-2835
www.mcrfmd.com

Communications Editor: Suzanne M. Hartung
Illustrator and Graphic Designer: Lynne Majetic, RN, BA

Saving Legs,

Saving Lives...

Peripheral Vascular Disease Made Simple

NICOLAS W. SHAMMAS MD, MS, FACC, FSCAI
Editor-in-Chief

and

Eric J Dippel, MD, FACC
Assistant Editor

with
Contributing Authors

Illustrator and Graphic Designer: Lynne Majetic, RN, BA
Communications Editor: Suzanne M. Hartung

Important Note:
Never Hesitate to Seek Medical Attention!

We hope and intend that this book will help you understand the nature of peripheral vascular disease and how to communicate more effectively with your healthcare provider.

This book - including any and all information, product information, data, text, graphics or other materials that may appear herein - is intended solely for general education and information purposes and is not intended to be used to make medical or health-related decisions without the involvement of healthcare professionals.

The information in this book is not a substitute for, nor does it supersede, professional medical advice.

If you are seeking medical advice, you should consult a physician or other qualified health provider. Never hesitate to seek medical attention!

To my wife, Gail, and my
children, Waheeb, Andrew and Anna,
for their unconditional love and
encouragement, and to my mom, Vera,
for her endless sacrifice and support.

Nicolas W. Shammas, MD, MS

This book is dedicated to my father,
who inspired me,
and to my family - Missy,
Tyler, Kyle and Molly -
who support me.

Eric J. Dippel, MD

Saving Legs, Saving Lives: Peripheral Vascular Disease Made Simple

Table of Contents

viii

Preface

Saving Legs, Saving Lives . . . Peripheral Vascular Disease Made Simple is a timely project that addresses an endemic but currently under-recognized problem in medicine. PAD (Peripheral Artery Disease), a disease of the blood vessels that supply the lower extremities, is likely to continue to increase in the future with the rise in obesity and diabetes. PAD leads to amputations and is associated with a high rate of cardiovascular death and strokes. Over the past several years there has been an exponential increase in peripheral vascular procedures that address the problem of PAD. The answer to fight this disease, however, is first and foremost in its prevention. In this book we address the diagnosis, prevention and treatment of PAD and invite our readers to play a key role in assisting in fighting this relentless disease that is costing our healthcare system billions of dollars and thousands of lives every year.

This book was written in question-and-answer format to help the readers go directly to the questions they have in mind. We do hope that it will be a valuable resource to every individual who reads it, providing accurate knowledge about PAD from prevention to treatment. Fighting PAD is a lifetime process with a clear desire for a disciplined lifestyle change to conquer harmful habits. We do hope that we have made it easier for our readers to be equipped with accurate information to move forward toward more healthful living.

The editors are indebted to the generous support we have
received to the Midwest Cardiovascular Research Foundation
(www.mcrfmd.com) in support of this project, specifically
from the Scott County Regional Authority, Genesis Health
System and Cardiovascular Medicine, PC. We are also
indebted to the tireless efforts of many individuals who
have made this book a reality by providing a high level
of expertise, passion and dedication. I would like to
acknowledge in specific our communication editor Suzanne
Hartung and our Medical Illustrator Lynne Majetic. We also
thank all our Foundation's staff for their dedication and hard
work and their support to this project.

Together we can save legs and save lives. Let the battle
begin!

Nicolas W. Shammas, MD, MS
Founder and Research Director
Midwest Cardiovascular Research Foundation

Chapter 1

What is Peripheral Arterial Disease and How is it Recognized?
Nicolas W. Shammas, MD, MS

What are the peripheral arteries?
The heart pumps blood into a series of blood vessels or "tubes" that we call **arteries**. These vessels deliver the blood that carries oxygen to various organs of the body. The arteries that supply all organs with the exception of the heart (**coronaries**) and the brain (**carotids**) are called **peripheral arteries**. Among the peripheral arteries are those that deliver blood to the abdomen, chest, arms, legs, kidneys and various other vital organs.

In contrast to arteries, the **veins** bring blood into the heart to be pumped into the lungs and get loaded with oxygen. Chapter 11 will address diseases of the veins.

You might hear about **peripheral vascular disease (PVD)**. This is a general term that describes diseases that affect both arteries and veins. The term **peripheral arterial disease (PAD)** describes diseases that affect the arteries only. This will be the focus of this chapter.

1

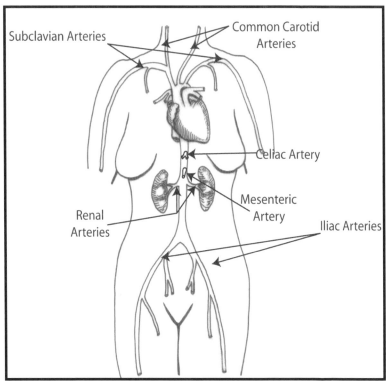

Figure 1. *Major peripheral arteries*

What does the term "disease of the arteries" mean?

Disease of the artery is a non-specific term but generally indicates build-up of plaque in the actual wall of the blood vessel. Plaque (or atherosclerosis) is a build-up of cholesterol, calcium, various blood elements and muscle cells under the lining of the artery. Generally, the artery accommodates the build-up by bulging outward to keep a wide opening for the blood to go through. However, when a plaque reaches 40% or so in severity, it starts to protrude inside the opening of the artery (***lumen***) and begins the actual narrowing process of the artery. This is commonly called **blockages of the arteries** or, as many people call it, **disease of the arteries**. Disease of the arteries, however, can be due to other factors, including **inflammation**, **infection**, **aneurysms** and others. For the sake of this book we will be focusing on diseases of the arteries that are related to blockages from **cholesterol build-up**, or **plaque**.

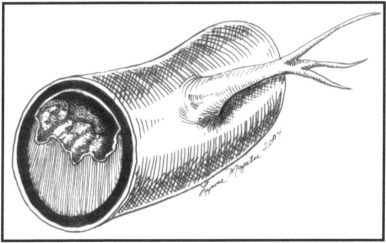

Figure 2. *Plaque build-up in an artery*

How common is Peripheral Arterial Disease (PAD)?

PAD affects 12-14% of the general population and becomes more prevalent with age, affecting up to 20% of patients over the age of 75. PAD also exists in conjunction with other diseases of the arteries, namely the **coronaries (arteries of the heart)** and the **carotids (arteries of the brain)**. Most people with PAD do not die of PAD itself, but rather of heart attacks and strokes. This is the reason why an aggressive screening for PAD is indicated to identify these high-risk patients and modify their increased risk. Patients with PAD sometimes can have no symptoms or they could be symptomatic. PAD symptoms consist of pain in the calf muscle when walking with resolution with rest (*claudication*) or *rest foot pain* at night when lying down with non-healing wounds or change in the color of the foot (*limb ischemia*). Limb ischemia is more serious and generally tends to increase the risk of amputation in these patients. The risk of dying from a heart attack or a stroke is higher in proportion to the severity of the disease in the lower legs. Therefore, preventive treatment in these patients is of paramount importance, and other chapters will address this issue in this book.

What is the natural history of PAD?

The natural history of PAD indicates that among patients with *claudication*, 7% will undergo lower-extremity bypass surgery, 4% major amputations, and 16% worsening claudication. Claudication is present in 5% of men and 2.5% of women over the age of 60. The rate of progression to advanced symptoms at rest or *gangrene* is estimated at 2.2% per year. However, nonfatal cardiovascular events (*heart attacks*, *stroke*) occur in approximately 20% over a 5-year period, and the 5-year mortality rate is estimated to be 30% (versus 10% in controls), of which 75% were cardiovascular deaths.

This natural history is very different from patients with advanced-rest symptoms or non-healing wounds on their legs. **Limb loss** is more prevalent in these patients, and the worse the symptoms, the more likely they will experience an amputation. In fact, patients with severe symptoms have a 28% chance to lose their leg at 6 months and 34% at 12 months. When all patients with advanced limb symptoms at rest are evaluated, the overall amputation rate ranges from 10-40%, with a mortality rate of 20% at 1 year, 40-70% at 5 years and 80-95% at 10 years.

Therefore, the goals in treating the PAD patient are: 1) reduce cardiovascular mortality in this high-risk population, 2) improve quality of life in severe claudicants, and 3) lower the chance of amputation in patients with limb ischemia as manifested by rest limb pain or *ulceration*.

Can a patient with PAD present as an emergency?

PAD patients can have the emergence of abrupt symptoms of rest foot pain, change in the foot color, and/or loss of sensation and motor function of the foot. The foot typically will have no detectable pulse and is painful. The vessel is typically occluded with a clot that suddenly forms in the arteries on top of an existing blockage. A patient that presents with sudden onset of lower foot pain, numbness and a change in the foot color needs to go to the emergency room immediately and will likely require an immediate treatment with a

5

procedure that opens the blockage in the artery and restore blood supply to the foot. Delays in going to the emergency room can lead to gangrene in the foot (***tissue death***) and likely loss of the foot or even the patient dying from these complications.

How can PAD be recognized?
PAD can be recognized either by a reduced pulse in the feet when examined in a doctor's office or by the symptoms a patient describes. A patient with discomfort in his or her hip or calf muscles when walking that improves at rest, or patient with rest foot pain when elevating the foot and the pain resolves when dangling the foot down, or patients with non-healing wounds on their legs are likely to have PAD. There are other reasons for a non-healing wound on the legs, but PAD has to be excluded in these patients. PAD is highly prevalent in a diabetic, and a low threshold to screen these patients is suggested. Also, smokers tend to be at high risk of PAD. A diabetic smoker will multiply his or her risk of PAD and other cardiovascular events such as stroke or heart attacks. On occasion, a patient with PAD presents with symptoms that are not typical and non-specific. If these patients have multiple risk factors, particularly diabetic or smokers, screening them for PAD is recommended. The presence of PAD is a strong indicator that the patient is at high risk of stroke or heart attacks. Testing to diagnose PAD will be discussed in a later chapter.

Chapter 2

Peripheral Vascular Disease
Eric J. Dippel, MD

What is Peripheral Vascular Disease (PVD)?
Peripheral vascular disease (PVD) is a term that describes blockages in the blood vessels that supply the entire body except the neck and head (called cerebrovascular disease) and the heart (called coronary artery disease).

Cholesterol not only clogs up the arteries of the heart, but it also clogs other arteries in the body. All of the arteries in the body are susceptible to this problem. The arteries to the neck are called the carotid arteries and they supply the head. When the carotid arteries become significantly blocked, patients are susceptible to stroke. This is explained more fully in Chapter 5.

The arteries to the kidneys, known as the renal arteries, also frequently become blocked. Typically, there are no symptoms associated with renal artery narrowing. However, since the kidneys are one of the organs that control your blood pressure, any sudden increase in your blood pressure might be a sign that your kidney arteries are becoming blocked.

Blockages can occur anywhere in the arteries to the legs. When this occurs in a mild or moderate degree, the most common symptom is claudication, which is a "tight" or "tired" sensation in the leg muscles that occurs with walking and is relieved with rest (see "What is Claudication?" below). When the blockages to the leg arteries become severe enough, then tissue in the leg begins to develop ulcers and die. If blood flow is not re-established promptly, then patients may require amputation of part of the leg.

What are the Risk Factors for Peripheral Vascular Disease (PVD)?

The risk factors for PVD are identical to the risk factors of coronary artery disease (CAD): high cholesterol, cigarette smoking, diabetes, high blood pressure, obesity, and a family history of vascular disease. Since our arteries in our bodies become blocked up over time, PVD typically gets worse as people become older.

Since the risk factors for PVD and CAD are the same, many patients have both problems at the same time. Patients with PVD that is uncontrolled are more likely to die from heart attacks and strokes rather than from blockages in their lower legs.

Among the above risk factors, smoking is the most hazardous for patients with PVD. Quitting smoking not only reduces the risk of further disease, but also can be one of the most important interventions that can be done to

8

reduce symptoms of pain in the lower legs.

How Common is PVD?

PVD is quite common, although it is frequently under-recognized and under-diagnosed. A simple analogy is: when grandpa walks to the mailbox and gets chest pain, he is referred to the emergency room. However, when grandpa walks to the mailbox and his legs get tired, he simply is told he is "just getting old."

There are millions of Americans who have PVD, yet only a fraction actually receives treatment. Furthermore, there are thousands of amputations performed in this country every year that might be prevented if blockages obstructing the blood flow to the leg were detected and treated early. There are over 12 million people in the USA who live with peripheral vascular disease, but fewer than 25% are being treated. A higher index of suspicion is necessary for both patients and physicians to adequately search for, diagnose and treat PVD.

What is Claudication?

Claudication refers to the symptoms of leg fatigue and cramps that patients with PVD describe when they exert themselves. This is typically described as a "tight" or "cramping" sensation in the calves, thighs, or buttocks that occurs with walking. Typically, this occurs at a very predictable time in walking. For example, after walking one to two blocks, a patient would have to stop and rest.

Leg cramps at night while sleeping are typically not due to PVD. However, foot pain at night, along with discomfort in the calves with walking a short distance, can be a sign of very advanced PVD that would require immediate attention.

Advanced lack of blood supply to the lower extremities can result in skin ulceration, non-healing wounds and infection and ultimately tissue loss and amputations. Dependent rubor and elevation palor are terms that describe advanced blockages in the arteries of the legs. When blockages are very severe, elevation of the legs leads to less blood supply to the foot that turns pale and when the leg is dangled down the foot turns red (gravity assisting the blood in reaching the feet). Patients sometimes complain of their feet and toes turning blue when dangled down. This is generally due to venous stasis, or pooling of the blood to the lower legs, rather than insufficient blood reaching the toes.

What are the Causes of Leg Pain?
Leg pain can be broken down into three major categories.

1. The first category are problems with blocked blood vessels and poor circulation. As described above, these symptoms of claudication occur with walking or exertion and are alleviated with rest. Patients can develop pain that occurs with rest only if the blockages are severe and the blood flow to the leg is extremely limited. Typically, if

this occurs, there are other findings, such as discoloration of the skin or ulcerations of the foot, that go along with resting pain from poor circulation.

2. The second major type of leg pain is due to problems with the bones and joints, such as arthritis of the knees, ankles, and hips. This type of pain is typically worse with standing and weight bearing on the joint. It may occur at rest and, not uncommonly, is improved with walking.

3. The third major type of pain is caused by nerve problems. For example, pinched nerves in the low back can cause sciatica pain which shoots down the hip and buttocks into the lower leg. This pain typically feels sharp and may be worse with certain positions. Another type of nerve pain is numbness and tingling of the feet that is frequently seen in diabetes. This has a sensation of "pins and needles" and may be present 24 hours a day.

What Tests Can be Done to Evaluate for PVD?

These tests can be broken down into noninvasive studies versus invasive studies. The simplest noninvasive study is simply by measuring the blood pressures in the arms and comparing it to the blood pressure in the legs. This is known as the ankle/brachial index (ABI). The blood pressure in the ankles should be roughly the same as the blood pressure in the arms. If the ankle blood pressure is significantly decreased, then this is evidence that there are blockages somewhere in the legs. Pictures of the arteries in the legs can be obtained through either a CT scan or an MR scan. While these images are similar, for technical reasons, the CT scan probably provides more accurate images. Doppler ultrasound can also be used to measure blood flow into the arteries. This test is most commonly used to monitor the adequacy of blood flow through bypass grafts, but also can be utilized to assess the flow to the native arteries. Invasive studies include the angiogram test. During this test, a catheter is placed in the arm or leg (at the groin level) under local anesthetic and contrast dye is injected through it to visualize the arteries.

What is the Treatment for PVD?
The two most important treatments for PVD are aggressive risk factor modification and a daily walking program. It is extremely important that the risk factors mentioned above be controlled to prevent these blockages from becoming worse over time. The most effective steps that patients can take to modify these risk factors are to stop cigarette smoking and lower their cholesterol, diabetes, and blood pressures to normal recommended levels.

Walking is very important to help maintain muscle tone, lower body weight, and develop better circulation to the feet. Patients should try and achieve a goal of walking 30 minutes a day, at least 5 days a week. There is one medication that has been approved by the FDA, called Pletal ® , that can help improve blood flow to the feet. Pletal has been shown to increase the distance patients can walk before they develop claudication. For mild claudication it is a very effective medication. It does not by itself, however, "dissolve" the blockages that are in the arteries, and patients with moderate-to-severe claudication frequently require procedures to open up blocked arteries.

What Types of Procedures Can be Performed to Open Blocked Arteries in the Legs?

Similar to the heart, arteries in the legs can be opened by using catheters with balloons and stents or by surgery to bypass the blocked vessel. Patients typically prefer balloons and stents because this is less invasive. This is called a percutaneous procedure, in contrast to the surgical one that requires a bypass. Percutaneous procedures significantly shorten recovery time with less discomfort, and the long-term outcome results are as good or better than surgery. Therefore, the first-line approach to opening blocked blood vessels in the legs should be with a balloon or stent if the blockage is amenable to this kind of therapy. If the artery cannot be successfully opened percutaneously, then surgery is an alternative.

What Risks are Possible with Angioplasty to the Legs?

Although angioplasty and stents are preferred to surgery, these procedures are not without risks.

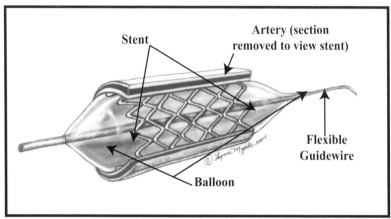

Figure 3. *Balloon mounted stent being deployed in artery*

Major complications can happen, although infrequently. The following is a list of the most important serious complications:
1. death (0.1%)
2. major bleeding (2-3%)
3. limb loss particularly in the patients with advanced lack of blood supply to the legs (1%)
4. kidney failure (1-10%) especially in the patient with heart failure, preexisting kidney disease and diabetes
5. early closure of the artery after as successful treatment that will require subsequent treatments
6. damage to the blood vessels and nerves at the puncture site (typically in the groin)
7. to a lesser extent, infections, strokes and heart attacks

What Risks are Possible with Surgery to the Legs?
Surgery to the legs can carry all of the above risks in addition to a longer recovery phase from

14

generally bigger wounds.

What is an Aneurysm?
An aneurysm is a "weakened" area of an
artery that is bulging out in the same way
that a garden hose may develop a bulge at a
weak spot. The danger in aneurysms is if they
become large enough, they can spontaneously
rupture. Aneurysms can occur throughout
the body but most commonly occur in the
main aorta that runs down through the chest
and abdomen. If an aortic aneurysm were to
rupture, this could be a life-threatening event.
Therefore, aneurysms are typically repaired
with surgery or more recently, with less invasive
stent grafting, prior to rupture.
Unfortunately, many times aneurysms do
not have any symptoms until they begin to
rupture. If your doctor suspects the presence
of an aneurysm on examination, further testing
can be ordered to evaluate the presence of
an aneurysm in you. Screening for aortic
aneurysms can be done using an abdominal
ultrasound or CT scan.

Why Do My Legs Swell?
Leg swelling, or edema, can be caused by a
number of reasons. Some of these problems
may be quite serious, while others are rather
benign and cosmetic. Swelling in both legs may
represent a heart or kidney problem, or a more
benign problem is incompetent valves in the
veins of the legs (varicose veins). Swelling in
one leg may represent a blood clot in that leg
or a blockage in the lymph nodes in the groin.
It is also common for a leg to swell after veins

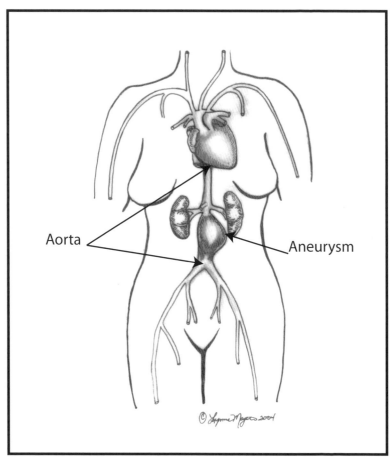

Figure 4. Abdominal aortic aneurysm

have been removed for coronary artery bypass grafting. Any new swelling of one or both legs should be evaluated by your primary care physician.

What is Abdominal Angina?
Abdominal angina is pain in the abdomen resulting from blockages to the main arteries that supply the guts. It typically presents itself with pain in the abdomen after eating

that cannot be explained by gastrointestinal pathology such as gallbladder disease or ulcers or inflammatory diseases. Blockages in those arteries called the celiac arteries or mesenteric arteries can lead to a reduction in the blood supply needed for digestion and transport of food to the body from the guts.

Patients typically experience predictable pain in the abdomen with food and weight loss. Cholesterol plaques cause a narrowing in these arteries similar to blockages in the neck, heart and legs. Treatment of these blockages can be done with either surgery or with angioplasty and stents. The diagnosis is best made by a CT angiogram or a conventional angiogram in the catheterization laboratory.

Generally, treatment of these blockages can lead to resolution of symptoms almost immediately after the procedure.

Summary: Ways We Can Reduce the Risks or Impact of Peripheral Vascular Disease (PVD)
1. Quit smoking
2. Walk at least 30 minutes 5 times per week
3. Maintain an appropriate body weight
4. Reduce blood pressure and cholesterol
5. Aggressively manage your diabetes with the help of your doctor and dietitian
6. Seek medical attention promptly if experiencing foot pain at night, along with discomfort in the calves when walking a short distance

This chapter was previously published in **Learn About Your Heart . . . Made Simple and Live Longer, Live Healthier**, *edited by Nicolas Shammas, MS, MD, Midwest Cardiovascular Research Foundation, Davenport, Iowa.*

Chapter 3

Diabetes: the Most Powerful Risk Factor of Peripheral Arterial Disease
Joseph E. Bergstrom, DO, CWS

What is Diabetes?
Diabetes is a chronic disease characterized by ***high blood sugar***, or ***glucose***. It is believed that approximately 24 million American adults have diabetes, and it is projected that that number will increase to 30 million by 2020. Unfortunately, up to a third of people with diabetes do not know that they have the disease.

Symptoms of diabetes, or that may indicate that you have diabetes, include ***frequent urination***, ***increased thirst***, ***delayed wound healing***, ***vision changes***, ***weakness***, ***fatigue*** and ***weight loss***. Most people with diabetes have no symptoms.

Diabetes is not a new disease. Physicians in ancient Greece described the disease and gave it the name diabetes, which means sieve, in reference to the large amount of urine that people with diabetes produce. The urine tasted sweet, or like honey, which is why ***diabetes***

mellitus is the proper term for diabetes related to high blood sugar.

Are there different types of diabetes?
There are four types of diabetes mellitus.

Type 1 diabetes occurs when the pancreas stops producing **insulin**. Insulin is a hormone that is needed to control the glucose or sugar level in your body. Type 1 diabetics need to inject themselves with insulin to keep their blood glucose controlled. Three quarters have people with Type 1 diabetes are diagnosed before the age of 18 years. Less than 10% of people with diabetes have Type 1 diabetes.

Type 2 diabetes is the most common type of diabetes, affecting 80-90% of people with diabetes. Type 2 diabetes is believed to be caused by a decrease in production of insulin by the pancreas in combination with insulin resistance.

Gestational diabetes occurs during **pregnancy**. This type of diabetes frequently resolves after delivery. A history of gestational diabetes is also a risk factor for developing Type 2 diabetes.

Diabetes can also be caused by **genetic defects in the production of insulin**, by the **use of certain medication** or by **other metabolic disorders**, such as **cystic fibrosis**.

How is diabetes diagnosed?

Diabetes is diagnosed by measuring your *blood glucose level*. A *fasting blood glucose* (no caloric intake for at least eight hours) of more than 126 mg/dL (7.0 mmol/L), usually on two separate days, is the most common method to diagnose diabetes.

Diabetes can be diagnosed in people that have the symptoms of *high blood glucose* (increased urination, increased intake of water and unexplained weight loss) and have a *casual blood glucose* of more than 200 mg/dL (11.1 mmol/L). Casual measurement means any time of day regardless of when you last ate.

Diabetes can also be diagnosed using a 2-hour oral glucose-tolerance test. A *fasting blood glucose* is performed, and if the result is less than 126, you will drink 75 grams of glucose dissolved in a liquid. This frequently tastes like cola or orange drink. Two hours later, another blood glucose level is checked. If the result is more than 200 mg/dL (11.1 mmol/L), then you have diabetes.

Your physician may also want to check a *hemoglobin A1c*, or *glycosylated hemoglobin* or sometimes just *A1c*, test. Hemoglobin is the molecule in your red blood cells that carries oxygen. The A1c site can bind with glucose in your bloodstream, and the percentage of the sites that are bound to glucose is measured. Because everybody has glucose in their blood, a hemoglobin A1c of less than 5.5% is considered normal. The hemoglobin A1c is usually ordered to monitor response to diabetic treatment, but is not recommended to be used to diagnose diabetes.

What is pre-diabetes?
High blood sugar (glucose) that is high but not high enough to meet the criteria to be diabetes is called **pre-diabetes**. There are two types of pre-diabetes: **impaired fasting glucose** and **impaired glucose tolerance**. Impaired fasting glucose is diagnosed when a fasting blood sugar is between 100 mg/dL and 125 mg/dL. A fasting glucose of less than 100 is normal. Impaired glucose tolerance is diagnosed when a two-hour glucose is between 140 mg/dL and 199 mg/dL. A two-hour glucose of less than 140 is normal. Both types of pre-diabetes are risk factors for future diabetes.

What are the risk factors for diabetes?
Risk factors for having diabetes include physical inactivity, a first-degree relative with diabetes, being a member of a high-risk ethnic population, having a baby weighing more than 9 pounds or having a history of gestational diabetes, having been or currently being treated for high blood pressure, having a low high-density lipid level or a high triglyceride level, having polycystic ovarian syndrome, severe obesity, age, or known cardiovascular disease.

Physical inactivity is less than 150 minutes per week of moderate-intensity exercise. **Moderate-intensity exercise** raises your heart rate to 50-70% of your maximum heart rate. Your **maximum heart rate** is calculated by subtracting your age from 220. For instance, if you are 50 years old, your maximum heart rate is 170. During moderate-intensity exercise, your heart rate should be between 85 and 119.

First-degree relatives are your parents, your siblings and your children. Aunts, uncles and grandparents are **second-degree relatives**. A first-degree relative with diabetes is a risk factor for diabetes.

Certain **ethnic populations** are at high risk of developing diabetes. These ethnic populations include **African American**, **Latino**, **Native American**, **Asian American** and **Pacific Islander**.

If you have **hypertension**, or **high blood pressure**, then you have a risk factor developing diabetes. Hypertension is a systolic blood pressure of more than 140 mm Hg or a diastolic blood pressure of more than 90 mm Hg measured on two separate days.

Abnormal lipids (parts of cholesterol) can also be risk factors for diabetes. A low level of high density lipids (HDL) is one abnormality. HDL is the good cholesterol, so a low level of less than 35 mg/dL (0.9 mmol/L) puts you at higher risk.

Triglycerides are part of **lipid metabolism**. A triglyceride level of more than 250 mg/dL (2.82 mmol/L) is associated with diabetes.

Women diagnosed with **gestational diabetes** are at risk of having diabetes. Also, women who have given birth to a child weighing more than 9 pounds are also at risk.

Women who have **polycystic ovarian syndrome** have a risk factor for diabetes.

Being **overweight** or **obese** is a risk factor for diabetes. Eight percent of people with Type 2 diabetes are overweight or obese and twenty percent of overweight or obese people will become diabetic. **Body mass index (BMI)** is used to determine if you are overweight or obese. You can determine your **BMI** by dividing your weight (in kilograms; 1 kilogram=2.2 pounds) by the square of your height (in meters). For example, a 1.5-meter-tall person who weighs 100 kilograms has a BMI of 44.4 (100 divided by 2.25). A BMI of more than 24.9 is considered overweight and a BMI of more than 29.9 is considered obese.

A history of **cardiovascular disease** is another risk factor for diabetes. Cardiovascular disease includes a **heart attack (myocardial infarction)**, **coronary artery disease**, **carotid artery disease** (severe narrowing of the arteries in your neck that supply blood to your brain), **abdominal aortic aneurysm** (widening of the largest artery in your abdomen), **stroke** or **peripheral artery disease**.

Age of more than 45 years of age is also a risk factor.

Should I be tested for diabetes?
Testing is recommended for all adults who are overweight (BMI of 25 or more) and have additional risk factors:
- physical inactivity
- first-degree relative with diabetes
- member of high-risk ethnic population
- women who delivered a baby weighing more than 9 pounds
- women with gestational diabetes
- women with polycystic ovarian syndrome
- high blood pressure (more than 140 mmHg systolic or 90 mmHg diastolic)
- on medication for high blood pressure
- HDL cholesterol less than 35 mg/dL
- triglycerides more than 250 mg/dL
- impaired glucose tolerance
- impaired fasting glucose

All persons should be screened for diabetes or pre-diabetes starting at age 45. If testing results are normal, screening should be repeated at least every three years.

What are the complications of diabetes?
Cardiovascular disease is the major cause of disability and death for people with diabetes.

Cardiovascular disease is usually a result of **atherosclerosis**, or narrowing of the arteries. Narrowing of the arteries around your heart is **coronary artery disease**. This can lead to **angina** or **heart attacks**. Narrowing of the arteries in your neck is **carotid artery disease** and can lead to **strokes**. Narrowing of the arteries in your legs is **peripheral arterial disease**. This can lead to **skin ulcers**, **gangrene** and **amputations**.

Diabetes can lead to damage of the kidneys, or **nephropathy**. **Diabetic nephropathy** occurs in 20–40% of patients with diabetes and is the leading cause of end-stage renal disease, which can result in dialysis or even death.

Vision problems are also common in people with diabetes. In **diabetic retinopathy**, the small blood vessels that supply the back of the eye, the **retina**, are weakened and leak. Diabetic retinopathy is the most frequent cause of blindness among adults aged 20–74 years. **Glaucoma** and **cataracts of the eye** also occur earlier and more frequently in people with diabetes.

High blood sugar also causes damage to **nerves**. **Peripheral neuropathy** is damage to the nerves in the limbs, especially in the feet. This nerve damage results in pain, tingling and the eventual loss of the ability to feel. The lack of sensation in the limbs leads to ulcers, foot sores and sometimes amputation. **Diabetic autonomic neuropathies** are also damage to the nerves caused by high blood sugars. Symptoms of these includes **resting tachycardia** (**fast heart rate**), **exercise intolerance**, **orthostatic hypotension** (a rapid drop in blood pressure when moving from supine to sitting or sitting to standing positions), **constipation**, **gastroparesis** (delayed stomach emptying), and **erectile dysfunction**.
26

Can diabetes be prevented?

Studies have shown that people with **pre-diabetes** can prevent developing diabetes by decreasing their body weight by 5-10% and exercising for at least 150 minutes of moderate activity each week, or preferably for 30 minutes every day.

For people with pre-diabetes and at least one other risk factor, the addition of the medication **Metformin** can also prevent diabetes. This was especially effective if the person had a BMI of 35 or more and was less than 60 years old.

What treatments are available for diabetes?

Diet and **exercise** are the cornerstones of treatment for diabetes. Studies have shown that 5-10% loss of body weight and moderate exercise for 150 minutes per week can lower glucose levels and delay the development of the complications of diabetes.

However, if diet and exercise are not sufficient to meet treatment goals, there are currently 14 oral medications and two injectable medications for the treatment of diabetes. These medications can be divided into three groups: those that increase insulin in the body, those that decrease the entrance of sugar into the body, and those that decrease insulin resistance.

Most people with Type 2 diabetes will be on the oral medication Metformin. Metformin increases the insulin sensitivity in the muscles and improves insulin function in the liver.

People with kidney disease should not take metformin.

Pioglitazone and **Rosiglitazone** also decrease insulin resistance. These medications also work in the liver and muscles, but also in the fat cells in the body. Because these medications can cause edema, they should be avoided in people that have **congestive heart failure**.

Sitagliptin works in the gastrointestinal tract to improve the function of insulin. Sitagliptin should be used cautiously in people that have kidney disease.

Acarbose and **Miglitol** are both **alpha-glucosidase inhibitors**. These medications work in the intestine and delay the absorption of glucose from digested foods, thus decreasing the amount of glucose in the bloodstream.

Colesevelam is a **bile acid sequestrant**, a medication that blocks the absorption of fat from the gastrointestinal tract, that also helps to decrease blood glucose level.

Nateglinide, **Repaglinide**, **Chlorpropamide**, **Glimepride**, **Glipizide**, **Glyburide** and **micronized Glyburide** all increase the secretion of insulin from the beta cells of the pancreas. This increase in insulin helps to lower blood glucose levels.

The injectable medications are **Exenatide** and **insulin**. Exenatide helps to block destruction of insulin in the gastrointestinal tract and thus prolongs its ability to lower blood glucose. Exenatide also decreases the sensation of being hungry, which helps to promote weight loss as well.

Insulin comes in multiple forms. Long-acting or basal insulin helps to lower fasting blood sugars throughout the day. Shorter-acting insulin helps to lower blood glucose right after eating. Frequently, people with diabetes will need to be on a combination of insulins to get adequate control of their blood glucose. The use of insulin requires frequent monitoring of your blood sugar to prevent **hypoglycemia**, or **low blood sugar**.

What are the treatment goals for diabetes?
The **American Diabetes Association** recommends the following as the goals of treatment of diabetes:

- A fasting glucose between 70 and 130 mg/dL
- A postprandial glucose of less than 180 mg/dL
- A hemoglobin A1c of less than 7.0%
- No episodes of hypoglycemia or low blood sugar
- Blood pressure of less than 130 mmHg systolic and less than 80 mmHg diastolic
- An LDL level of less than 100 mg/dL if no cardiovascular disease
- An LDL level of less than 70 mg/dL if you have cardiovascular disease
- An HDL level of more than 40 mg/dL if you are a man

- An HDL level of more than 50 mg/dL if you are a woman
- A triglyceride level of less than 150 mg/dL
- Receive an annual influenza vaccine
- Receive a pneumococcal vaccine
- If you smoke, stop

Chapter 4

Smoking: The Next-Most-Powerful Risk for Peripheral Arterial Disease

Shawna K. Duske, RN, BSN, ARNP

How many people are still smoking?
Smoking worldwide continues to rise, with an estimated 1.3 billion people who smoke. Most of these individuals live in developing countries where estimates are as high as 1 in 2 male smokers. In the United States, the number of adults smoking has been decreasing for several decades. In the 1960's, over 40 percent of adults smoked on a regular basis. Current estimates indicate that this number has declined to 19.8 percent in adult smokers. States that grow *tobacco* tend to have higher percentage of adult smokers; for instance, 28% of adults in Kentucky smoke tobacco. Utah has the lowest rate of tobacco use at 12%. The number of *teenage smokers* has not dramatically changed over the last several years.

Why do people smoke?
People start smoking for a variety of reasons, including peer group acceptance, belief in the tobacco companies' advertisements, or just as an experiment. Those persons who

31

start smoking before the age of 18 are more likely to continue smoking longer, and most wish they had never started. People continue to smoke because their body has become addicted to the substances found in cigarettes, particularly nicotine. The body's requirement for **nicotine** cues a person to smoke in order to function comfortably and avoid the side effects of **nicotine withdrawal**. Nicotine is a strong psychoactive drug comparable to **amphetamines**, **cocaine** or **opiates** for producing euphoria, or a state of well-being. This euphoria is related to both the amount of nicotine absorbed into the body and the rate that absorption occurs. This euphoria is highly addictive.

Nicotine withdrawal can begin in as little as two hours. Besides the loss of the euphoric effect, withdrawal can also cause a **depressed mood**, **insomnia**, **irritability**, **anxiety**, **difficulty concentrating**, **increased appetite** leading to **weight gain**, and **restlessness**.

What are the complications of smoking?
There is not an organ system that is not affected by cigarette smoking. There is an increased incidence of **oral and esophageal cancers** compared to non-smokers. Those persons who smoke have an increased incidence of **pulmonary disease**, including **COPD**, **chronic bronchitis** and **lung cancer**. **Tobacco use** is an independent risk factor in the development of **coronary artery disease** and other **vascular disease** of the body including **stroke** and **PVD**.

32

The effects of cigarette smoking are estimated to be responsible for greater than 10 percent of all *cardiovascular deaths* worldwide. Smoking increases the risk of *peptic ulcer disease* as well as *diabetes*. In women who smoke there is an increased incidence of *infertility*, *spontaneous abortion*, and *premature menopause*. Smoking accelerates changes in bone density in both men and women, leading to *osteoporosis*. The incidence of *bladder cancer* is also increased in those individuals who smoke. Finally, smoking has been shown to age persons by 10-15 years; thus, smokers tend to have more *changes in the skin*, making them appear older than their stated age.

What are the effects of secondhand smoke?
Secondhand smoke is the term applied to the involuntary exposure of tobacco smoke from the smoking of others. As people became more aware of the systemic effects of smoking, as well as the increased incidence of cardiovascular disease and cancers in individuals who smoke, studies soon followed documenting the effects of secondhand smoke.

Studies have shown that *children exposed to secondhand smoke* have an increased incidence of *ear infections*, *respiratory illnesses* including *asthma* and *pneumonia*. For women who smoke during their *pregnancy*, the developing baby is exposed to the same amounts of tobacco as that of an active smoker. There are more *stillbirths* associated with smoking during pregnancy. In addition, the birth weight of the baby is usually lower and there are more **oral facial clefts**, as well as possible associations with **congenital heart disease**. Experts estimate that each year 50,000 deaths are related to cardiovascular disease and nearly 5,000 deaths related to lung cancer are due to direct exposure to secondhand smoke.

How does smoking worsen PAD?

Smoking greatly increases the risk of developing **atherosclerosis** (**clogging of the arteries**). Some studies indicate this may be as high as 50 percent in current smokers compared to non-smokers. The number of years smoked and the number of pack of cigarettes may also correlate to the progression of disease. There are probably multiple factors involved in the development of atherosclerosis since smoking does not appear to affect all individuals in the same way. Studies indicated that smoking is associated with an adverse effect on **lipids** as well as with **insulin resistance**. In addition, some of the chemicals found in cigarette smoke damage lipids, resulting in the formation of potentially dangerous particles in the bloodstream. Tobacco use produces an increase in **heart rate** and **blood pressure**. Research also indicated that smoking damages the lining of blood vessels and may reduce the elastic properties of the vessels. Smoking also affects the body's ability to prevent **clots**.

Is smokeless tobacco safe?

There is no such thing as a safe tobacco.

34

Individuals who smoke *low-tar cigarettes* or *low-nicotine cigarettes* generally smoke more cigarettes and inhale longer to avoid withdrawal of nicotine. In addition, individuals who use *smokeless tobacco* are exposed to a greater incidence of *oral and esophageal cancers*.

How can I quit smoking?

Most people who smoke know the health hazards of smoking and wish to quit. On average it takes up to four attempts for a smoker to remain tobacco-free. Realizing the health and social benefits of *smoking cessation* outweigh the benefits of smoking is essential to success. After quitting smoking, the risk of cardiovascular disease associated with smoking is reduced in 2 years. After 10 years, the risk is nearly equivalent to a person who has never smoked.

Persons who have been successful in quitting smoking state the importance of identifying a plan as well as identifying the triggers that causes them to smoke. Realize when you smoke and formulate a plan to include activities that can replace smoking. Avoid activities that increase your desire to smoke. It is important to involve as many friends and family as possible in your decision to quit smoking. Pick a quit date and mark the day with a celebration to increase your commitment to *quitting smoking*. Involve your health care provider in your decision to help you choose the best method that will be successful for you. There are many programs available including *nicotine* replacement therapy, *group smoking-cessation programs*, *self-help programs*, and *medications*.

What medications are available to help me quit?

There are numerous over-the-counter *nicotine-replacement medications* available, as well as two prescription medications to help people quit smoking.

Nicotine polacrilex is available as a gum or a lozenge. When the gum is chewed or the lozenge absorbed through the lining of the mouth, nicotine is released into the blood stream. This nicotine should not be swallowed, as it will cause gastric upset. The nicotine polacrilex forms come in two- or four-milligram strengths and should be used for no more than six months. This nicotine replacement medication has approximately a 15% rate of abstinence at one year.

Transdermal nicotine patches are another method of nicotine replacement. A patch is placed on the skin, and nicotine is released into the venous blood system in a continuous manner while the patch is in contact with the skin. Abstinence rates at one year are approximately 15%, similar to the nicotine polacrilex system.

A *nicotine nasal spray* and a *nicotine inhaler* are also available as nicotine replacement systems. A nicotine inhaler is a plastic holder into which cartridges containing nicotine vapor are delivered into the lining of the mouth when inhaled. The nicotine is not actually inhaled, just absorbed into the lining of the month. Frequent puffs are required to avoid nicotine withdrawal symptoms. One cartridge may last one to two hours, and an individual may need 6 per day. The length of recommended use is 6 to 12 weeks, with abstinence rates being equal to other nicotine replacement substances.

The antidepressant **bupropion** is marketed as **Zyban** to help people quit smoking. The recommended dose is 150 milligrams daily for three days, then 150 milligrams twice daily for at least 12 weeks. Abstinence rates are approximately 23% at one year after discontinuation of bupropion.

Varenicline is a prescription medication that has been shown to help people stop smoking. This is marketed as **Chantix**. Chantix is dosed 0.5 milligrams daily for three days, then 0.5 milligrams twice daily for the next four days, then 1 milligram twice daily for at least 12 weeks. This medication has more side effects than the other therapies, but is twice as effective as bupropion. Bupropion and varenicline are not nicotine products, thus nicotine replacement products may be used with these medications for a short period of time to enhance your commitment to smoking cessation.

Studies have shown that combining behavioral therapy with medication therapies increases the success rates more than either treatment alone.

Are there other resources that can help me?

There are many resources available to help you stop smoking.

Your **physician** or **health care provider** is a good place to start. Most physicians have received training in the best methods to encourage their patients to stop smoking.

Your community also has resources. **Hospitals** and sometimes **churches** will often have support groups to help people quit smoking. The **American Cancer Society**, the **American Heart Association** and the **American Lung Association** all have on-line resources and may have an office in your community that will be able to provide information on the steps to stop smoking.

Many states have developed programs to help people stop smoking. The programs are funded by the money that **tobacco companies** were required to pay to settle the claims against them. Your local **health department** should be able to direct you to these programs.

Chapter 5

Peripheral Arterial Disease: Symptoms and Management

*Peter P. Toth, MD, PhD, FAAFP,
FCCP, FAHA, FACC
Director of Preventive Cardiology
Sterling Rock Falls Clinic
Sterling, Illinois*

What is Atherosclerosis?
Atherosclerosis, or "*hardening of the
arteries*," can occur in any portion of the
cardiovascular system. In recent decades,
much research has focused on the development
of atherosclerosis in the arteries of the heart
(**coronary arteries**).

Atherosclerosis leads to the formation of
blockages that reduce **blood flow** to such
critical tissues as the **heart**, the **brain**, and the
muscles in your legs. If the blockages become
large and severe enough, then the delivery of
blood decreases to the point where the **tissues**
nourished by affected blood vessels die due to
the lack of oxygen. When this occurs, people
experience such complications as **heart attack**,
stroke (or a "**brain attack**"), or the **loss of a
leg**.

In this chapter, we will explore the symptoms,

diagnosis, and treatment of atherosclerosis in the lower extremities. This is also known as **Peripheral Arterial Disease**.

What is Peripheral Arterial Disease (PAD), and how does it relate to Atherosclerosis?

Peripheral arterial disease is a highly dreaded form of atherosclerosis because it can be quite disabling. As patients develop blockages in the arteries of their lower extremities, oxygen delivery to the muscles and skin of the leg progressively decreases. The **oxygen deficit** in **leg muscles** can manifest as **leg pain** with such forms of exertion as **walking** or **running**. This leg pain is called **claudication**. It is typically relieved by rest and recurs when the person resumes walking.

Where does Claudication occur?

Claudication can occur anywhere along the length of the leg, from the buttocks to the foot and toes. The location of pain generally correlates with where along the length of the leg vasculature an **atherosclerotic plaque** is developing. Physicians and patients alike can mistake pain in the buttocks and thigh as being secondary to **arthritis** in the hip or knee, **lower-back problems**, **phlebitis** (pain stemming from inflammation in a vein), **muscle injury** or **inflammation**, or **neuropathy**. Classically, pain occurs in the calf; however, it can also manifest as hip, thigh, knee, ankle and foot pain.

What are some symptoms of Claudication?
The pain is typically dull and achy and can be accompanied by rapid onset of lower-extremity fatigue. Symptoms can also be described as a *heaviness*, *numbness*, or *tightness* in various distributions of the leg.

Because Peripheral Arterial Disease can also lead to reduced blood perfusion of the skin, patients can present with a variety of other signs and symptoms that should prompt consideration of *lower-extremity atherosclerotic disease*. *Discolored skin*, due to *tissue congestion* and reduced *vascular drainage*, can occur. If various regions of the skin have inadequate oxygen delivery, *skin ulcers* and *erosions* can develop that are quite resistant to healing. *Hair follicles* in the skin may die, resulting in *hair loss* most prominently along the calf and lower thigh. The leg may feel cool due to reduced blood flow.

What is the most significant danger of PAD?
Peripheral arterial disease must be taken seriously. The most dread complication of this disease is the development of *gangrene* in the toes or feet, necessitating *amputation*. Patients can also require amputation below the knee and above the knee. This, of course, is catastrophic as the patient is left with *disability*, both physically and emotionally.

Another complication of peripheral arterial disease is *critical limb ischemia,* which can be a surgical emergency. In the setting of critical limb ischemia, an **atherosclerotic lesion** has either ruptured or has suddenly increased in volume, leading to a potentially catastrophic reduction in the capacity to deliver oxygen to the leg. Emergency intervention must often be undertaken to save the extremity and prevent the need for amputation.

Which patients are most likely to have PAD?

Unfortunately, the two groups of patients most seriously impacted by Peripheral Arterial Disease are patients with **diabetes mellitus** and those who **smoke**.

However, it is important to understand that other patients also can develop peripheral arterial disease. Other risk factors for Peripheral Arterial Disease include **abnormal cholesterol levels**, **hypertension**, increasing **age**, chronic **kidney disease** and **obesity**. There appears to be a slight preponderance of this disease among men, but this **gender** difference appears to be disappearing as more women smoke and more women become diabetic.

What is the relationship between diabetes and PAD?

A devastating complication of poor blood sugar control in the setting of diabetes mellitus is the development of severe Peripheral Arterial Disease. It is always extremely sad when a diabetic patient begins having to have one or more toes, a foot or a leg amputated. This results in considerable disability and loss of **quality of life**.

42

How is PAD diagnosed?

A simple test can help to determine if you have Peripheral Arterial Disease. An **ankle brachial index** (**ABI**) simply measures blood pressures in your ankles and arms. If the ABI is less than 0.9, this pretty much cinches the diagnosis. The diagnosis can be confirmed with a **lower-extremity angiogram**. If a patient develops severe pain or is on a course to develop critical limb ischemia, consideration must be given to reestablishing **blood flow** to the leg. This is typically done by defining the anatomy of the blood vessels in the leg with either a **CT angiogram** or a **magnetic resonance angiogram**. These are extremely sensitive tests that can help to define the precise location of a blockage as well as its relative severity.

How is a blockage treated?

A critical blockage can be treated in one of two ways. The first is to perform **angioplasty** and **stenting**. This is the same procedure that cardiologists perform in heart blood vessels. A lesion is identified and the blood vessel is opened with a **balloon**. The blood vessel is then propped open with a stent. The second is to perform a **bypass surgery** around a blockage. If a patient has stable disease in that it is classified as being either mild or moderate, then medical treatment with aggressive **lifestyle modification** is the most appropriate therapeutic approach.

What types of lifestyle modification can patients make to manage PAD?

Anyone diagnosed with Peripheral Arterial Disease is assumed to also have *coronary artery disease* (i.e., it is by definition a coronary artery disease risk equivalent). Consequently, your doctor may elect to do a *stress test* or a *coronary calcium score* with a *CAT scan* to more precisely evaluate whether or not you have evidence of heart disease. Follow his or her advice on this, as it may be life-saving.

Patients are entered into a *monitored exercise program* through a hospital or clinic. Increasing the amount of time devoted to *walking* and *exercise* helps to improve arterial vessel wall function and is associated with progressively less claudication. Patients feel better as they exercise more, and symptoms almost always improve. This can also result in *weight loss* and reductions in *insulin resistance* and improvements in *blood sugar*.

In addition, it is critical to quit *smoking*. There is no question that a smoker with Peripheral Arterial Disease can expect his or her disease to worsen fairly rapidly. Do not wait to quit smoking. Once you lose toes, a foot, or a leg, you cannot get them back. If you need medication to quite smoking, talk to your doctor about *nicotine gum* or *patches*, **Chantix** or *Wellbutrin* therapy, or *counseling*.

If you have diabetes or are *prediabetic* (i.e.,

insulin-resistant), it is important to lose weight and get your blood sugars under control. **Blood glucose** when elevated is highly toxic to your blood vessels. Weight loss typically works best when it is done in collaboration with a **dietitian**.

What types of medication are available to treat PAD?

In addition to lifestyle modification, **drugs** play a prominent role in the management and treatment of Peripheral Arterial Disease. You should try to get your **low-density lipoprotein cholesterol** (**LDL-C**) to less than 70 mg/dL. **Statins** (**Lipitor**, **Crestor**, **Zocor**, **Pravachol**) are the preferred means by which to do this. **Statin therapy** is associated with reduced frequency of claudication in patients with peripheral arterial disease.

Among diabetic patients, the drug **fenofibrate** has been shown to reduce risk for lower-extremity amputation by 38% over 5 years. Blood pressure should be reduced to less than 130/80 mm Hg.

Among patients with Peripheral Arterial Disease, multiple studies have shown that **ACE inhibitors** (**ramipril**, **lisinopril**, **enalapril**) confer long-term benefit. Your **good cholesterol** (the so-called **HDL**) should also be raised above 40 if you are a man and above 50 if you are a woman. Your **blood triglycerides** (**blood fats**) should be kept at a minimum below 150 mg/dL.

If you have Peripheral Arterial Disease, you should also take **aspirin** every day (81-325 m/dL, depending on you specific circumstances. You should discuss this with your doctor. If you have more advanced disease or if you have coronary disease and have been stented, then your aspirin should be supplemented with **Plavix**, which is associated with increased long-term benefit (reduced risk for heart attack, stroke, and **death**). Another medication that has been shown to be helpful is **Pletal** or cilostazol. Pletal therapy has been shown top increase the distance a patient with peripheral arterial disease can walk without precipitating pain. Remember, the more you walk, the better you will do in the long run (yup, pun intended!).

The beauty of aggressive therapy is that for many patients, the severity of their disease actually can improve or regress. Therapy is also associated with less need for **arterial revascularization**, a lower incidence of amputation and disability, and it is unequivocally associated with reduced risk for heart attack, stroke and death.

I think we all agree these are favorable outcomes. Approximately 12 million people in the United States have Peripheral Arterial Disease. This is likely an underestimate. If you are having symptoms that suggest the presence of Peripheral Arterial Disease, get it checked out. Your life (and legs) can depend on it.

Chapter 6

The Role of Exercise in the Treatment of Peripheral Arterial Disease
Conway Chin, DO

Exercise for the treatment of a medical condition should be done under the guidance and input of your physician. The following questions will go over some basics regarding the role of exercise in beginning to add this treatment for improvement in your overall health and quality of life.

Why is exercise helpful?
Exercise is very important in the treatment of ***peripheral arterial disease***. Exercise, especially ***aerobic exercise***, will help the ***muscles*** in our body, particularly the arms and legs, become more efficient with the energy, oxygen and nutrients provided by the body. As one exercises, the muscles will be able to do more work with less oxygen and nutrients. As a result, there will be less demand on the **heart**, **lungs** and ***circulation system***. Therefore, one will be able to do more things with less ***fatigue***. So even if the peripheral arterial disease does not improve in a person, exercise will allow us to be able to do more things for ourselves in caring

47

to our daily needs and adding quality to our lives.

Who should exercise for the treatment of peripheral arterial disease?

Everybody, whether they have peripheral arterial disease or not, should perform aerobic exercise. The aerobic exercise should be tempered based on one's own circumstances and schedule. It is helpful to exercise with a partner to provide supervision and motivation. It will allow a person to be able to re-start exercise more easily if they take a break due to a vacation or other circumstances.

What type of exercise should be done?

Aerobic exercise is the optimal exercise treatment of peripheral arterial disease. Aerobic exercise involves repetitive activity of large muscle groups. **Walking**, **cycling** and **jogging** are the most common examples of aerobic activity. Other types of exercise, such as **strengthening**, **endurance building** and **stretching**, are helpful for our overall condition but are not as uniquely helpful to the treatment of peripheral arterial disease as aerobic exercise. Aerobic exercise can help us **lose weight** and **improve our overall sense of well-being**.

The aerobic exercise should start with a warm-up to gradually loosen the body to avoid injuries. After aerobic exercise of up to 20 minutes, a cool-down exercise can be done to gradually transition the body to a more normal routine. As one's conditioning improves, then a person

48

can extend his or her aerobic activity to greater than 20 minutes. It is important not to over-extend oneself too far as that may cause injury and discomfort that would discourage a person from continuing aerobic exercises over the long term. Exercise should be done with comfortable footwear that does not aggravate the foot, the legs or the back during the repetitive aerobic activity. It is important to consider one's safety when performing exercises as the goal is to improve health and not to add more problems to their clinical condition. The exercise intensity should be high enough to make it difficult to speak several words in a sentence before becoming too short of breath to continue talking.

Where should exercise to treat peripheral arterial disease be done?
Exercise can be done anywhere that allows a person to have repetitive activity. This could be on a stationary bicycle or a treadmill in an enclosed setting. This could be done at home or at a fitness center. If the weather and surroundings permit, then a park or a mall could also be a good place for exercise. It is recommended to have a partner or to exercise in a group setting to watch each other for problems. It is also likely to be more fun to exercise with others and can provide other important interactions, such as *socialization*.

When should exercise for the treatment of peripheral arterial disease occur?
As exercise should be done no matter what one's condition, then the amount will depend on one's

schedule. Exercises can be done daily, every other day or three times a week. A minimum of three times a week is recommended in order to obtain benefit from the aerobic exercise in the treatment of peripheral arterial disease. In order to avoid injury and boredom, many people cross-train with other types of exercise activities to provide a long-term commitment to a regular exercise routine. This may involve changing the place of exercise, changing the type of exercise (such as stretching or strengthening) and varying the intensity and frequency of the exercise.

How hard should one exercise to obtain benefit in the treatment of peripheral arterial disease?
One gauge is to measure the amount of exertion one feels that he or she is putting out with the repetitive aerobic exercise. This would involve one's own measure on the level of **_exertion_**. For example, on a scale of 1 to 10 (with 1 being the easiest and 10 being the hardest), one may shoot for an exertion level of a 7 to sustain over 20 minutes to achieve a significant benefit in improving one's aerobic condition. This can be tempered by the amount of **_pain_** experienced during the exercise activity. In this situation, pain is not a safe or advisable target to shoot for. Pain can put increased strain on the heart and lungs and can cause a person to have higher chances of serious problems. As a result, if one is having pain, one should stop the aerobic exercise activity and **_rest_** until the pain subsides. If the pain does not subside, then one

should seek help from either one of the exercise partners, who can then gauge if medical attention is needed.

The role of exercise is very important in the treatment of peripheral arterial disease. It provides treatment even if the peripheral arterial disease does not improve. It can improve **quality of life**, promote well-being and allow a person to function more independently in their daily routine. Always ask a physician for guidance in implementing exercise for the treatment of peripheral arterial disease. Further healthcare providers can be of assistance, such as an *exercise specialist*, *physical therapist* or a *cardiac nurse*.

Chapter 7

Diseases of the Blood Vessels of the Head and Neck
Eric J. Dippel, MD

What Are the Blood Vessels That Lead to the Brain?
There are four major blood vessels that go to the brain: two *carotid arteries* and two *vertebral arteries*. The two carotid arteries are in the front part of the neck; these can actually be felt pulsating adjacent to your Adam's apple, just below the angle of the jaw. The two vertebral arteries go to the back of the brain and run in the bony portion of the spine. All four arteries connect with each other in the brain. *(See Figure 5.)*

What is Carotid Artery Disease (CAD)?
Carotid arteries, like the other arteries in the body, can become clogged with cholesterol over time. The risk factors that cause these blockages include: high cholesterol, cigarette smoking, diabetes, high blood pressure, and family history. When the carotid arteries become severely narrowed, this can lead to decreased blood flow to the brain, which can subsequently lead to a *stroke*.

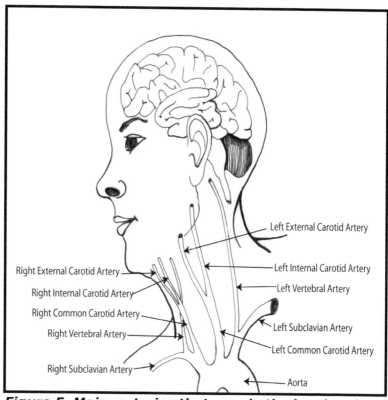

Right External Carotid Artery

Right Internal Carotid Artery

Right Common Carotid Artery

Right Vertebral Artery

Right Subclavian Artery

Left External Carotid Artery

Left Internal Carotid Artery

Left Vertebral Artery

Left Subclavian Artery

Left Common Carotid Artery

Aorta

Figure 5. Major arteries that supply the head and brain.

What are the Symptoms of Carotid Artery Disease?

Carotid artery disease is not associated with pain in the neck or headaches. When the carotid arteries become significantly narrowed, the blood can actually be heard "whooshing" through the blockage when a physician listens to the neck with a stethoscope. This noise is called a ***bruit***. Some patients might experience chest pain and/or dizziness.

54

What are the Risk Factors for Carotid Artery Disease?

The risk factors for carotid artery disease are the same as for a stroke:

1. Hypertension (high blood pressure)
2. Diabetes
3. A genetic tendency (family history)
4. Prior stroke or TIA
5. Lack of exercise
6. Poor diet
7. Obesity
8. Uncontrolled stress
9. Excess consumption of alcohol
10. Use of certain drugs that can weaken the heart muscle

How Can a Person Prevent Blockage in the Carotid Arteries?

The buildup of cholesterol, or **atherosclerosis**, in the carotid arteries occurs for the same reason cholesterol builds up in other arteries of the body. In fact, many patients that have coronary artery disease (CAD) or **peripheral vascular disease** (PVD) also have carotid disease. Aggressive modification of the risk factors that cause atherosclerosis will prevent the buildup of cholesterol in the arteries. This includes stopping smoking, lowering your cholesterol, controlling diabetes and high blood pressure, maintaining an ideal body weight, and getting regular exercise.

What Kinds of Tests Can Diagnose Carotid Artery Disease?

The simplest test is merely listening to the neck

with a stethoscope for a bruit. Some times, however, bruits may be difficult to hear. A more accurate noninvasive test is a **carotid Doppler**, which is simply an **ultrasound** of the blood flow through the neck. **CT scanning** and **MR scanning** can also be helpful in providing three-dimensional images of the carotid and vertebral arteries. Finally, the "gold standard" is an **angiogram**, which is an invasive test where a catheter is inserted in the groin and threaded up to the carotid and vertebral arteries. Contrast dye is injected through the catheter and x-ray movie pictures are taken of the arteries in the neck.

When Should a Person Have a Procedure to Open the Neck Arteries?

Whether or not carotid arteries should be treated with a procedure to open them up depends on several factors. One of the primary factors is whether the patient has had a prior symptom, such as a **stroke** or **TIA**, and the second major factor is the degree of **stenosis**, or narrowing in the artery. In combination, these findings have provided a framework for who should have a procedure to open the arteries versus who should simply continue on medical therapy to prevent further buildup of cholesterol.

How Can Blocked Arteries in the Neck Be Reopened?

Historically, the primary way to open up the carotid arteries is with surgery. This procedure has been performed for approximately 50 years and involves a surgeon cutting open the artery, scraping out the plaque, and sewing the artery back together. This procedure is known as a **carotid endarterectomy (CEA)**. Within the past few years, however, technology has evolved to the point where now the arteries can be opened up with a balloon and a **stent** via a catheter inserted through the groin under minimally invasive techniques. Recent data comparing carotid stenting versus surgery suggests that in certain high-risk groups of patients, stenting appears to be superior to surgery. Ongoing studies are being conducted to evaluate the most procedures for lower-risk patients.

What is an Aneurysm?
An **aneurysm** is a weakened segment of an artery that is bulging out, similar to the way a garden hose will bulge out at a weak point. The problem with aneurysms is that they are prone to rupture, which will cause bleeding in the brain and a stroke. Unfortunately, however, most

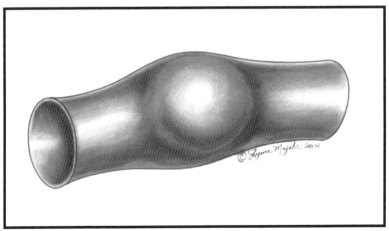

Figure 6. *Aneurysm*

people do not know that they have an aneurysm in their brain until it ruptures, because they typically do not have any symptoms beforehand, other than possible non-specific headaches. Aneurysms are usually a genetic problem, so if there is a family history of aneurysms, it would be worthwhile to be screened for one. *(See Figure 6.)*

How Are Aneurysms in the Brain Treated?
The traditional way to treat aneurysms in the brain was by surgery to clip the aneurysm sac. However, with recent advances in cardiac procedures, it is now possible to thread a small catheter up the artery from the groin into the brain and place small coils inside the aneurysm. The advantages of using the catheters are that the skull does not have to be opened and the recovery time is significantly less.

Summing Up . . . .
If you smoke, stop. Eat healthfully, maintain an appropriate body weight, get plenty of exercise. If you have high blood pressure, get it under control with a combination of weight loss, healthful eating, exercise and medication, as prescribed by your doctor. If you have a family history of aneurysms, get screened.

*This chapter was previously published in **Learn About Your Heart . . . Made Simple**, edited by Nicolas Shammas, MS, MD, Midwest Cardiovascular Research Foundation, Davenport, Iowa.*

Chapter 8

Nonhealing Wounds on Your Feet: The Need for Aggressive Treatment
Dr. Matthew Wilber, DPM

What is so special about your feet?
Your **feet** are very unique instruments. They contain 28 **bones**, each with multiple **muscles**, **nerves**, complex **arterial** and **venous networks**, as well as a **skin structure** that is unique for the entire body. All of these components within your foot function together to help you walk, run and jump as you participate in your daily activities.

Your feet are also capable of very high-functioning activities like dancing. Your feet represent the body part that is farthest from the brain. The brain is connected to your feet through a very advanced nervous system that allows the brain and feet to communicate with each other during our daily activities. These communications help regulate **muscle function**, **reflexes**, **blood flow** and **perspiration**.

They also serve a protective function by allowing the body to sense light and firm pressure, hot and cold, sharp and dull, vibration and position sense. **Position sense** is the body's ability to determine where it is in open space and maintain balance. An example of this would be walking on a rocky hillside. The brain would be able to determine the slope of the hill and the contour of the ground by processing messages sent from the nerves in the feet. The muscles in the legs and feet would then act to maintain balance after receiving messages from the brain. This back-and- forth communication takes place in a fraction of a second.

What can you do regularly to take care of your feet?

Maintaining good *hygiene* and *daily inspection of the feet* are recommended by multiple professional organizations, including the *American Podiatric Medical Association* and *American Diabetes Association*. *Inspection of the feet* should be done daily to look for any *calluses* or *corns*, *foreign objects*, *cuts*, *scrapes*, *reddened areas*, irregular *moles* or *freckles* and any unusual appearance to the *toenails* and nearby *skin*. Moles and freckles can present in a variety of colors, shapes and sizes. If present, these should be watched for changes in color, shape, size and the presence of flaking or bleeding. If any of these findings are noted, you should contact your physician.

Keeping the skin smooth and supple is ideal but often requires the use of powders and moisturizers such as creams and lotions. Occupational and recreational activity levels as well as climate changes can be challenging factors in maintaining smooth supple skin. Bathing the feet with soap and water should be performed daily and allows time for inspection. A hand-held mirror placed on the floor is a good tool for visualizing the bottom of the feet. It is important to dry between the toes to avoid developing the dark, moist environment that bacteria and fungus prefer.

Reddened areas can indicate that shoes do not fit appropriately, alteration of blood supply to the affected area, presence of an underlying disease process or an injury to the foot. Injuries can include insect or spider bites, foreign body penetration (splinters), small cuts or a result of blunt force. Sprains and strains can also result in redness and bruising of the foot and ankle, requiring monitoring by yourself and/or a physician until resolved. Wearing shoes that are of appropriate width and length can help avoid many problems that can affect the feet. Poor-fitting shoes, whether too big or too small, can result in increased risk of hammertoes, bunions, neuromas, calluses and ingrown toenails.

Regular trimming of toenails and calluses, if present, are simple maintenance activities. If you are unable to perform this on your own, a podiatrist or nursing service is often available to assist in this important measure of regular foot care. This is another good time for foot inspection.

Wearing clean shoes and socks every day is good practice to maintain foot health.
What is a wound?
Technically, a *wound* is any violation or breach

of the skin or layers beneath it. The skin consists of the outer epidermis and the inner dermis. Both the **epidermis** and **dermis** contain numerous layers. These layers cover the subcutaneous tissues where hair follicles, sweat glands and blood supply are located. Deeper still includes muscle, tendon and bone.

A wound can violate the body in a superficial manner where only the epidermis or outer layers are injured. Partial-thickness wounds involve both epidermis and dermal levels, and full-thickness wounds penetrate into the subcutaneous layer possibly extending to muscle, tendon and bone.

Wounds can be acute or chronic. **Acute wounds** typically will include blisters, stings or bites, lacerations, puncture wounds, gunshot wounds, open fractures or those associated with sustained direct pressure resulting in an ulceration. **Chronic wounds** more often are referred to as acute wounds that have not resolved in the expected time frame while under care or those that have not resolved due to failure of regular care to be initiated.

How does your body respond to a wound?
In the medical journals, it is generally accepted that there are 4 phases of wound healing.

- Initially, a period of **vasoconstriction** or **contraction of the blood vessels** to diminish bleeding at the site of injury takes place.

- Over the next 1 to 4 days, an ***inflammatory response*** to the wound is generated by the body to bring a variety of cells from the blood and tissues to fight infection, remove foreign materials and begin the repair process.
- The third phase, ***proliferation***, involves new blood vessel growth, tissue repair and growth in order to repair the wound defect. This typically takes place from days 5-21 after the wound began.
- Finally, the ***maturation/remodeling*** phase begins. This generally involves strengthening and reorganization of the former wound bed. The greatest amount of activity in this phase takes place from 6 to 12 months, but this phase can last up to two years following closure of the wound. Once the wound has fully remodeled, the resulting scar is at most only 80% of the tissue's original strength and elasticity. Depending on the location of the wound and its original cause, this diminished strength requires protection of the site in the future to prevent recurrence.

What factors most commonly cause wounds of the lower leg and foot?

Far and away the most common cause of lower extremity wounds is ***neuropathy***. Neuropathy results in the lack of the body to feel forces that would normally cause pain and those forces supplying excessive pressure leading to tissue breakdown.

Neuropathy is the cause behind lower-extremity wounds 53% of the time. This is followed by trauma, neuro-ischemic, venous stasis, pressure ulcers and gangrenous changes.

Neuro-ischemic wounds result from diminished feeling combined with poor blood supply.

Stasis wounds are a result of pooling of venous blood in the legs resulting in swelling and accumulation of toxins in the tissues resulting in wounds or ulcers of the lower legs.

Pressure ulcers can be the result of poor fitting shoes, poor fitting braces, prolonged bed rest and excessive standing or walking.

Gangrenous ulcers are primarily due to a focused loss of blood supply to an area, resulting in **tissue death**. These factors may be involved with an underlying disease. **Diabetes mellitus** is a common cause of peripheral neuropathy that primarily affects the lower legs and feet. Diabetes can also be associated with diminished circulation. It can affect both large and small blood vessels, resulting in chronic or acute deficiency of blood supply to the lower legs or feet. A wound that is present as result of diminished circulation and peripheral neuropathy in the diabetic patient can be very difficult to treat.

Other less common but notable causes of wounds include **infection, connective tissue diseases** such as rheumatoid arthritis and extended **radiation therapy**.

64

Why is aggressive treatment necessary for all wounds?
Wounds that are left untreated or those that are not immediately recognized are at greater risk for potentially severe complications. These complications include *soft-tissue infection*, *bone infection* and potential for loss of part or all of the foot or even *amputation* of the leg.

Infection can become so severe that it may even be life-threatening. International statistics indicate that there is a lower-extremity amputation every 30 seconds worldwide. Following a major lower-extremity amputation, nearly half of these patients die within a 3-year span and 60% within 5 years. Over 40% of these amputees have an amputation of the other lower leg within the first 3 years of the first amputation, and nearly 60% have this second amputation within 3-5 years of the first surgery.

Further statistics support the need for amputation prevention through aggressive wound care. These include findings that if amputation is performed secondary to loss of or diminished blood supply, the patient has up to a 33% chance of second limb loss within 3-5 years and up to a 45% chance of fatal heart attack within one year. If the patient has had a lower-extremity amputation and the ongoing presence of poor lower extremity circulation, there is a 41% chance of death from fatal heart attack within 3 years. Furthermore, if the amputation is combined with poor circulation and diabetes mellitus there is nearly a 50% chance of death from fatal heart attack within 3 years. These statistics are relative to the fact that if a patient is found to have peripheral arterial disease, up to an 80% likelihood exists that this patient also has central arterial disease affecting the heart and adjacent arterial structures. Only **pancreatic cancer** and **lung cancer** patients have a greater chance of death within 5 years from time of diagnosis than for a patient that has peripheral arterial disease and history of a lower-leg amputation.

The bottom line is that aggressive wound care must be performed in every case and at all times in order to prevent amputation.

What are the "costs" of a diabetic foot wound?

Diabetic foot wounds are expensive to both the patient and health care system. Hospital costs average between $50,000-100,000 per wound admission. In the United States more than 90 million disability days per year are attributed to diabetes. The estimated total cost of diabetes in the United States last year was $218 billion. The total cost for type I diabetics was estimated at $15 billion per year and $160 billion for type II diabetics.

Estimates were also made for those yet to be diagnosed with diabetes, $18 billion; women who temporarily develop diabetes during pregnancy, $636 million; and an increasingly common condition called pre-diabetes, $25 billion.

Ulcers affect 15-20% of all people with diabetes. They are present in 20% of all hospital admissions associated with diabetes. People with diabetes are 15 times more likely to experience an amputation. Foot wounds are the number one reason for admission to the hospital among people with diabetes. Approximately 90% of all lower-extremity amputations are a result of failure to treat these wounds. Diabetics who develop foot wounds are 56 times more likely to require hospitalization and 154 times more likely to require amputation of part or all of the foot.

On a brighter note, in the United States, non-traumatic diabetic lower-extremity amputations decreased from a high of 84,000 in 1997 to 75,000 in 2003.

What role does nutrition play in the wound-healing process?

Nutrition is a very important aspect of wound healing. When a patient presents to a doctor's office with a wound, performing a *nutritional screen* is part of the initial therapy process.

Nutrition includes appropriate water balance in the body to avoid *dehydration*, *dietary balance* of proteins, carbohydrates and fats, as well as recommended daily supplementation of *vitamins* and *minerals*. Vitamins A, B, C, E and K are required for effective wound healing, as well as   the minerals zinc, iron, copper, magnesium, calcium and phosphorus. Vitamins and minerals are important in cellular function and transport. Deficiencies in vitamin and/or mineral levels can affect all 4 phases of wound healing. Simple blood testing can reveal water balance, protein levels and vitamin and mineral levels.

Testing can also determine the protein level as well as *albumin*, *pre-albumin* and *transferrin* levels. Albumin is a blood protein that is often decreased if the patient is protein-deficient or *malnourished*. Pre-albumin is a blood transport protein. It has a shorter lifespan in the blood stream and is therefore more likely to indicate short-term changes in nutritional status whether to assess malnutrition or to see if nutritional therapy is helping. Transferrin levels are also very sensitive indicators of protein deficiency.

A doctor or dietitian should be consulted for appropriate *nutritional therapy*. Without professional assistance, it is possible for patients to take in excess water, protein, vitamins and minerals, resulting in potentially harmful effects on organs and other tissues in the body.

Why are the first four weeks of wound treatment important?

Several studies have shown that the first four weeks are a reliable predictor for how the wound will heal in the first 12 weeks and in some studies as much as the first 24 weeks. In other words, if the causes or maintaining factors of the wound are not addressed initially, the wound will most likely linger or worsen. These factors

68

include **blood supply**, **infection**, **pressure relief**, **swelling of the legs**, **management of underlying disease** and **nutritional status**. There are many other factors, but these are of primary importance.

Recommendations are that if the wound has not improved in the first four weeks despite efforts, more advanced therapy should be initiated. Wounds that have a more severe prognosis, such as those with poor circulation, infection or significant deformity, need to be addressed with aggressive and advanced therapy initially. People who eventually go on to heal their wound often show an 80% reduction in the wound surface area within the four weeks of treatment. On the other hand, those people who have delayed healing or do not go on to heal show only a 25% reduction in wound surface area within the first four weeks.

What is debridement and why is it important?

Debridement is a procedure performed on a wound to remove all nonviable tissue including **callus**, **foreign debris**, **soft tissue** and **bone**, if necessary. Debridement is performed to remove tissue at the cellular level as well. This helps remove inactive cells, stimulate active cells to participate in the wound-healing process and remove bacteria within the wound. Debridement is most commonly performed in the clinical setting but is also performed regularly in the operating room.

Good, thorough debridement is the cornerstone of wound management. The wound will not heal if dead tissue and foreign debris are not removed. During the debridement process, the surgeon is able to explore the wound for any pockets, tunnels, hidden **infection**, foreign matter or deeper **dead tissue**. If any pockets or tunnels are noted, they need to be aggressively opened and cleaned until the remaining tissues appear healthy and viable.

There are multiple debridement techniques that can be utilized by the physician. **Sharp debridement** can be performed with a scalpel, scissors or device called a **curette** that resembles a small ice cream scoop. There are prescription **topical enzymes** that gradually digest the dead tissue. The upside to these enzymes is they are often non-painful; however, they do need to be applied daily in most cases. **Ultrasound** and **high-pressure water-driven devices** are also available tools for debridement. These devices have been developed more recently and often allow debridement to be performed with less pain during and after the procedure. These devices can be used in the clinical setting or the operating room.

Larvae of the **Greenbottle fly** are very beneficial in performing pain-free debridement. These larvae are very efficient in digesting nonviable/dead tissue in the wound. The fluids emitted by the larvae have activity against numerous bacteria and help stimulate healthy

70

tissue growth. This type of debridement needs to be performed by experienced personnel and monitored very closely.

Manual debridement is performed by hand and includes some techniques we have just discussed. This is often done on a weekly basis to remove any callus build-up or other nonviable tissue that develops in order to continue stimulating the wound to heal. Sometimes debridement can be very extensive in that it may require primary **amputation** of a small or large portion of the foot in order to locate a healthy wound margin. It is often difficult to understand that by making a wound larger, improved healing can be promoted. But if clean margins are obtained throughout the wound during debridement, this is indeed the case.

Why is an acute wound preferable to a chronic wound?

An **acute wound** is a wound that has occurred recently. The body typically is in the process of mounting a healing response to this wound through the wound phases described previously. Once **vasoconstriction** or decreased bleeding is achieved, the body delivers a variety of blood cells and growth factors to the wound site. As the process continues, new blood vessel growth, cellular cleaning of the wound and new tissue growth take place. Eventually cells migrate across the wound bed, providing the cells necessary to form a new layer of skin. As mentioned above, this is primarily **scar tissue** that undergoes extensive remodeling over the next one to two years. In the absence of infection, poor blood supply and continued pressure on the wound site, this process has a good chance to heal the wound.

A **chronic wound** develops from an acute wound that has been neglected or has not responded to initial care. Chronic wounds also develop from failure to recognize the underlying cause. For example, if a wound has a diminished blood supply, the chances of this wound healing are significantly decreased. The same could be said for a wound that is affected by ongoing **infection**, repetitive or continuous **pressure**, or unrecognized underlying **disease state** such as **diabetes mellitus** or **malnourishment**.

In addition to addressing these potential underlying causes, another way to convert a chronic wound to an acute wound is through **debridement**. Debridement allows the physician to remove "sleeping" or inactive cells. This also helps remove any bacteria that may have colonized the wound. A wound can be colonized with bacteria without actual infection of the wound taking place. This colonization can create a "**bioburden**" for the wound, which interferes with normal cellular processes involved in the four phases of wound healing, thus allowing the wound to become chronic due to delayed healing. Debridement essentially restarts the healing process by creating a healthy, bleeding wound bed. This starts the wound-healing phases over again at the **vasoconstrictive** stage. If the body is functioning ideally the presence of growth factors, new blood vessel and tissue growth will ensue.

How can pressure be removed from an ulcer on the foot?

There are many ways to remove pressure from a **foot ulcer**. The **total-contact cast** remains the gold standard. This is a specialized cast that fits snugly around the foot and lower leg to remove pressure from the sole of the foot. Minimal underlying padding is utilized. This cast is constructed utilizing a mixture of plaster and fiberglass or just fiberglass. It cannot be applied to an infected wound or a wound where there is bone exposure. It is often changed weekly and, if no complications develop, can be utilized for extended periods of time on this weekly interval. Due to insurance coverage limitations for this cast, other off-loading techniques have been developed.

A custom-fit **offloading boot** called a **CRO walker** is probably the next closest relative to the total-contact cast. This boot has a firm, two-piece outer layer and is lined with a multi-density, soft offloading material. As this name indicates, it can be utilized for walking in a limited fashion. It can also be removed for dressing changes and showering daily if desired. Adjustments are often made to accommodate for occasional swelling. This is a moderately expensive boot but is very durable and the liner is replaceable.

An **ankle-foot orthotic**, or **AFO**, is also made from a custom cast of the patient's leg and foot. This is a stabilizing boot that has a multi-density insole for offloading of the foot, but this does not have the ability of a cast or CRO walker to relieve pressure from the bottom of the foot.

Other less-expensive walking boots are available, including the **CAM walker**, **neuropathic walker** and **DH walker**. A hybrid offloading boot is called an **instant total-contact cast** (**ITCC**). This essentially is the use of a CAM walker, neuropathic walker or DH walker that is wrapped in place either with an Ace wrap or layer of fiberglass. This assists the patient in maintaining offloading measures because it cannot easily be removed by the patient. None of these boots is a custom fit but can be effective in offloading as long as the patient understands that these boots are not meant for regular activity levels. Other offloading techniques include custom shoes and custom insoles that are accommodated to protect certain areas of the feet, surgical shoes with custom padding, diabetic accommodative shoes and heat-moldable inserts.

Of course, the very best offloading technique is to have no weight whatsoever on the foot. This is often not feasible for patients who lives alone or have to care for themselves and family members. Offloading is a crucial and challenging need for wound healing. This often has to be modified to fit the patient both literally and figuratively. For instance, if the patient has a significant amount swelling in his or her leg, a cast that fits snugly has a twofold problem.

1. The first is that if the patient were to swell even more this could lead to constriction of the foot and leg, resulting in acute **decreased blood supply**. This could even result in **gangrene** of the extremity.

2. The second problem can be if the swelling reduces under the compression from the cast, the cast is suddenly very loose and can piston up and down on the leg, leading to development of new pressure points and possibly new wounds. Therefore, in the case of a swollen extremity, the cast may need to be changed more often if the swelling decreases and checked regularly to see if it has become too tight.

What can be done to manage swelling of the lower extremities?

Swelling of the extremities is also known as **edema**. An older identifying term is **dropsy**. This can be a very complicating problem in managing wounds. It is often a principal factor behind the development of **venous stasis wounds**. Stasis often results from inadequate valves in the veins of the lower extremity, leading to pooling of blood in the venous system. Since the venous system carries toxins out of the extremities, this pooling process can result in increased venous permeability, allowing the toxins to seep out of the veins into the surrounding tissues. The body then forms an inflammatory response to these toxins, resulting in further increased swelling and redness. As the condition progresses, water blisters can form on the skin, developing into oozing sores on the legs that can rapidly progress into ulcers and are often very painful.

To avoid this process, **compression therapy** is needed. One way to manage edema is through **compression stockings**. Typically a graduated compression stocking is best. This supplies a varying level of compression from the toes to at least the knee if not up to the upper-thigh level. Other simple techniques to reduce edema include a **low-sodium diet**, **elevation of the legs** when sitting and **exercise**.

Elevation of the legs is best when placed above the heart level. A general goal is to perform this twice daily, for 30 minutes in the morning and 30 minutes in the evening.

Exercise is also a fantastic technique for reducing edema. The veins in the lower legs function primarily when squeezed by the muscles of the calf. Therefore, if one is exercising, these veins are intermittently compressed by this muscle action, mobilizing some of the static fluid. **Diuretics** are available naturally and by prescription. Prescription diuretics, which need to be monitored closely by the physician, are helpful in reducing edema that affects the lower legs and the central body cavity.

Some insurance plans cover **edema pumps**.
These pumps supply sequential pressure
from the foot to the upper leg, gradually
squeezing fluid out of the extremity. All
means of compression should be monitored
by a physician. It is necessary to be aware
of the **arterial pressure** in the leg so that
compression therapy does not exceed the
arterial pressure, resulting in loss of blood
supply to the limb.

**What kind of skin-grafting options are
available for wound treatment?**
There are numerous **skin-grafting options**
available to treat challenging ulcerations of
the lower extremities. The best option has
long been considered an **autograft**, which is
harvested from the patient's own body and
transferred to the desired defect. This is usually
called a **split thickness skin graft**. The
problem with this procedure is that creates
a second surgical site on the patient. If this
patient already has difficulty healing wounds,
creating a second wound needs to be considered
very carefully. If the patient's own skin is not
adequate or if the patient cannot tolerate the
surgical procedure itself, human tissue can be
cultured, grown and applied to these extremity
wounds. Two of these grafts are commercially
available. One is primarily **epidermal tissue**
while the other is primarily **dermal tissue**.
Both can be applied in sequential layers. These
are living grafts and are grown from the cellular
level. The cells are harvested from human
foreskin and are meticulously treated so that

77

no immune properties or disease is passed to the recipient. They contain growth factors and cellular elements that help stimulate healing once applied to the wound. When a person donates his or her body to science or more directly registers as an **organ donor**, the skin can be harvested, cleansed of immune properties and presence of any disease. Portions are then dried and sterilized. These grafts can be utilized on recipient wounds merely by reconstituting them in water. These grafts have no living cells but retain microscopic passageways and tunnels for new vessel growth and cellular migration into the wound defect. These grafts come in the form of variable-sized sheets and a liquid form that can be placed into deeper tunneling wounds that have been cleaned of dead tissue and bacteria. Since this particular graft is recognized as "self," the wound often will have very little scarring if it successfully heals. This graft can be placed internally as well. It has the ability to take on the form of the tissue where it is placed. It is a very strong and versatile graft.

Xenografts are grafts that come from species other than humans, including pigs, cows and horses. These grafts are often utilized for their **collagen** content. Collagen is a very strong fiber that is present in most tissues in the body. These grafts help set up a latticework into which the recipient's tissue can grow. All graft options fall into the advanced category for wound-healing tools. These grafts can only be utilized once blood supply has been optimized, infection has been treated, the wound relieved of pressure and any underlying disease controlled or least stabilized. Failure to do so will ultimately result in failure of the graft.

What is negative pressure wound therapy? *Negative pressure wound therapy* is the controlled application of **subatmospheric pressure** to a wound by utilizing electrical pump. This subatmospheric pressure has been shown to increase local blood flow, thus enhancing blood supply to the tissues in and adjacent to the wound. This increased local blood supply also increases the oxygen content to the wound. The negative pressure is essentially applying suction to the wound. In doing so it also helps reduce edema, protect the wound from bacteria and promote new tissue growth.

The machine commonly is referred to as a **wound VAC** or a **vacuum-assisted closure device**. Because it is completely portable, it can be utilized both in the hospital and on an outpatient basis. The drainage that is collected from the wound is held in a small canister contained within the device. The portable unit runs on a battery when taken outside the home and is simply plugged into a wall socket to recharge overnight. Before utilizing the VAC, the wound must be debrided of all nonviable tissue. The VAC can also be utilized in conjunction with skin grafting to help secure the graft and remove underlying fluid that can cause graft failure. This is another advanced tool but can be utilized as soon as the wound is prepared appropriately, as discussed previously.

The device is very quiet as long as an adhesive seal covering the wound is not leaking. If the seal is weakened or lost, a small alarm system will sound on the device, alerting the patient. A special sponge is applied into the wound and covered with the adhesive seal, and a small tube connects the wound to the portable unit. Several types of sponges are available to address wounds of varying depths and sizes. The wound VAC cannot be utilized on infected wounds or a wound with underlying bone infection.

Because the sponge and seal only have to be changed three times weekly, the expense of daily dressing changes is reduced as well as the human handling of the wound, thus reducing introduction of bacteria. Due to its universally accepted success, most insurance plans will cover this unit.

What role does hyperbaric oxygen therapy play in wound healing?
Hyperbaric oxygen therapy (*HBOT*) is another very useful tool to achieve wound healing. The treatments apply a higher level of oxygen in the bloodstream that can be delivered to the wound site if circulation is adequate to the wound. This is a very strictly regimented aid to wound healing in that there are only 13 indications approved for its use. In 2003, hyperbaric oxygen therapy was approved for

wounds that are caused by diabetes, have been treated conventionally for more than 30 days and have a depth that extends to tendon or bone in the presence of infection.

When utilized for wound care, hyperbaric oxygen therapy is rarely the sole mode of treatment for the wound. It can also be utilized in conjunction with failing skin grafts and flaps, as well as for those patients who recently have undergone an angioplasty or stenting procedure to improve the circulation to their lower extremities to aid in wound healing. Typical treatment times are 90 minutes in length and occur 5 days a week.

Hyperbaric oxygen therapy has also been shown to improve the body's immune response, improve bacterial killing ability and promote new blood vessel growth. The increased oxygen content stays in the body for 2-4 hours following treatment.

Typically a patient would undergo 20 treatments initially. The patient is assessed with a **_transcutaneous oxygen-measuring_** machine after 12-15 treatments to see if increased oxygen content is maintained during therapy. These test results are compared to a similar transcutaneous oxygen measurement taken prior to treatment. If no improvement is noted, treatment is often discontinued. If increased blood oxygenation levels are maintained, then treatment can continue. The sessions are monitored closely by a certified hyperbaric technician as well as an overseeing physician.

The chambers in which hyperbaric treatments take place are large, ***mono-place chambers*** or **multi-place chambers**. The patient is able to watch television, read the newspaper or watch a DVD movie while in the chamber. The mono-place chambers are large, non-confining chambers were the patient can recline or rest in the seated position.

Take care of your feet!
Careful, systematic foot care and prompt attention to all wounds are essential to good health and quality of life.

Chapter 9

Varicose Veins and Chronic Venous Insufficiency (CVI)
Richard Sadler, MD, FACS

Fundamental Concepts
Chronic venous insufficiency (CVI) is one of the most prevalent diseases in the United States, being approximately four times more prevalent than ***coronary artery disease***. However, because of its very slow onset and insidious course, the end stage serious portion is not reached for many years, lulling both the practitioner and the patient into a sense of complacency or resignation. To understand the problem and the treatment options, it is first necessary to understand how the venous system works.

How many veins are in the legs?
The veins of the lower extremity are divided to three anatomic sections. The ***deep veins***, which are matched with their named arteries, run deep within the leg and the muscle compartments and carry approximately 90% of the blood flow from the legs back to the heart. The ***superficial veins***, which lie just underneath the skin, carry approximately 10% of the blood. A small portion of blood is returned between communicating veins between the superficial and deep system, called ***perforator veins.***

How does blood move up the legs?

Much like other upright animals, in humans the blood in the veins makes its way to the heart when the human is in the upright position, aided by two mechanisms.

The first is the muscles of the calf, which form the **venous pump**. The contraction associated with walking actually forces blood from the superficial system, as well as the deep system, and pushes it up the veins towards the heart, similar to a water pump. This pump mechanism is initiated with walking, and it is effective for approximately 30 seconds after cessation of walking until gravity takes over and the blood pools within the veins.

The second key mechanism uses a series of valves within the superficial and deep venous system, which allows blood to progress towards the heart but not fall back or have retrograde flow when the human is standing, but not walking. These valves are the most common source of problems causing chronic venous insufficiency.

Why are leg veins vulnerable to gravity?

The column of blood within the veins are similar to a column of water in any type of upright pipe, the best analogy being a water tower supplying water pressure to a town. The fluid collects in the legs and will stay there for a prolonged period of time until either a change of position or initiation of the calf muscle pump allows the blood to drain out. **Venous insufficiency** (or *varicose veins*) can be caused by abnormal pressure of blood at the ankle level, deep vein obstruction, sometimes caused by injury or disease, deep vein reflux where the valves of the deep systems are involved, congenital malformations where the veins has developed in a dysfunctional way, or pump failure where the patient is unable to or cannot utilize the calf muscle.

How do patients with varicose veins feel?
The symptoms associated with vein disease actually follow a rather orderly progression, and these are the basis of the **American Venous Form Classifications**, called **CEAP**. It was initially a research tool to classify and organize research into vein disease. It has, in fact, become the clinical standard. The first letter, "C," is the most useful portion and it is given a numerical value.

- **C0:** A person who has **no vein disease** and is otherwise normal.

- **C1:** This is the **beginning of vein disease** often characterized by what is called **"spider" veins** or small **violaceous reticular veins** forming small networks underneath the skin.

- **C2:** *Varicose* – Veins have now become enlarged and visible; they vary in size and position or are sometimes associated with major vein insufficiency, or are sometimes isolated. In any event, they are the start of the symptomatic **chronic venous insufficiency**, and they represent failure of blood to return normally and are the clinical evidence of the beginning of **venous hypertension**.

- **C3: *Edema* –** The collection of fluid in the subcutaneous tissue is seen when the venous pressure from the standing column of water exceeds the diastolic pressure of the arterial system. The column of fluid then seeps into the surrounding tissues and in between the cells, causing a chronic swollen edematous state.

- **C4: *Skin changes* –** When the venous hypertension is long-standing and the subcutaneous edema is chronic, eventually there is **fibrosis** in the small microvessels and tissues of the subcutaneous tissue and skin, which then results in **eczema**, **redness**, **itching**. Fibrosis occurs in both small microscopic arteries and veins, as well as scar tissue and collagen deposition. This becomes a hardened, rigid type of swelling often called **"brawny" edema**. Left untreated, the skin changes will not be reversible, although the changes can be arrested with the appropriate treatment.

- **C5: *Healed ulcer* –** Once the skin has become damaged enough it eventually breaks down due to a microscopic **hypoxia** and **ischemia** of the skin itself. As these cells die, they form small ulcers sometimes leading to large ulcers. Ulcers sometimes heal, and the subsequent scars are the basis of the C5 classification.

- **C6:** This is the presence of an *active ulcer* from the skin breakdown as mentioned above and is the most advanced form of chronic venous insufficiency. When this occurs, a treatment is mandatory, and left untreated, the prognosis is grim because the ulcer will continue to enlarge and coalesce with time, ultimately resulting in circumferential loss of skin around the leg at which point amputation becomes a possibility.

Why do varicose veins look so similar in so many people?
A thorough understanding of the vein disease requires understanding of the patterns typically seen.

The *intravenous trunks* are those larger vessels that run vertical, with orientation starting at the ankle and moving to the hip. These major trunks include the greater and lesser *saphenous veins*, which are in the subcutaneous compartment, and the deep veins paired with their arteries, as mentioned above.

The majority of chronic venous insufficiencies occur because of a *truncal reflux*. The superficial system, particularly the *greater saphenous vein*, is involved in approximately 85% of the saphenous vein or chronic venous insufficiency. The *lesser saphenous vein* is involved in approximately 15% or a combination of both.

Sometimes the truncal system remains intact; however, there are large varicosities noted along the lateral posterior portion of the thigh, and these are typically the **anterior accessory saphenous veins** or the **vein of Giacomini** around the leg. Although not truncal in origin, they have the capacity to enlarge significantly, participate actively in **venostasis** and are often quite symptomatic.

Rarer types of reflux occur in the **pudendal** or **pelvic circulation**, which flow from the upper-inner thigh downward, as well as pure, isolated **perforator veins**, which communicate between the superficial and deep compartments.

Can I inherit varicose veins? Are there other causes?

Risk factors for chronic venous insufficiency are multiple, but most important is **heredity**. When both parents have chronic venous insufficiency, their children have approximately 90% risk of having it also. When one parent has venous insufficiency, there is a 25% chance that the male offspring will have the same problem and a 62% likelihood that females will.

Excluding injury or extrinsic changes to the vein, the propensity of women to have this problem is greatly associated with **pregnancy**. Although, for years it was thought that the weight gain and increasing pelvic pressure of pregnancy was a source of problems, it is much more dependent on the very high levels of progesterone. The progesterone has smooth muscle, relaxing qualities, which are necessary to prevent uterine rupture and to allow normal uterine expansion. This same effect, however, is also true on the vascular system, and although the arterial system has the ability to recover from the stretched or dilated shape, the venous system has a much sparser muscular layer, resulting in a permanent dilatation of those veins which are congenitally already susceptible to disease. Once the valves of the superficial system becomes stretched and incompetent, the beginning of the venous hypertension starts with the reflux or retrograde flow, putting downward pressure on more veins, again causing them to become insufficient, resulting in a vicious cycle which leads to the classic full-length truncal insufficiency associated with severe **venous reflux**.

How are varicose veins treated?

There are several ways to treat varicose veins. The easiest and often the most overlooked approach is simply called **vein hygiene**. Here the patient must take action to minimize the increased pressure and reflux, thereby relieving the pressure on the tissue. This includes **weight reduction**, **smoking cessation**, regular **exercise**, and **elevation of the legs** when ever possible to allow passive venous return toward the heart. It is critical for the practitioner to remind the patient that appropriate elevation means keeping the distal leg or ankle at or above the level of the heart. Fluid can only flow passively downhill on a negative gradient. Therefore, passive drainage can only occur when the legs are elevated higher than the level of the heart. An often overlooked but extremely useful technique to assist this is to have the patient sleep in a head dependent manner all night long. This is easily and cheaply accomplished by using 4"x 4" blocks under the foot of the bed so that the entire bed frame is tilted slightly downward relative to the patient's head. This creates a small but consistent gradient, allowing passive flow all night long. Patients report rapid and significant resolution of their swelling with this technique, which is of minimal cost and essentially zero risk. Although other treatments are necessary, this type of vein hygiene is a fundamental part of all treatment programs and should be encouraged.

The second mainstay of care is **moisturization of the skin**. Once skin changes have started to occur, the breakdown then results in loss of normal sweating and oil-producing mechanisms, which cause breaking of the skin, cracks, and fissures. This then becomes a portal for infection, resulting in **ulceration** and sometimes **cellulitis**. **Good skin care**, which includes prevention of cuts and abrasions from shaving, as well as moisturization, is important.

Why do I have to wear stockings?
The mainstay of non-surgical treatment has been extrinsic compression with **gradient compression stockings**. Modern stockings or

compressive devices are manufactured with a built-in gradient so that the highest pressure is at the ankle, corresponding to the area of highest pressure due to hydrostatic forces. These stockings provide a constant pressure to advance the blood uphill, against gravity, and enhance return of the blood to the heart.

Although the stockings are relatively cheap, patients sometimes do not use them because of their chronic discomfort and more importantly because of the manner in which they must be used. Properly applied, gradient compression stockings need to be applied quickly upon arising from the bed so that the fluid does not have a chance to accumulate in the legs. The stockings need to be worn most of the day and should not be removed until the patient then retires for sleep. It is sometimes successful to remove the stocking if the patient is anticipating a vigorous or prolonged exercise using the calf muscle pump, but again it should be emphasized that the cessation of walking for as little as 30 seconds will allow the hydrostatic forces to again overcome normal tissue pressure and begin the swelling process.

Can I do anything besides use the stockings?

Because **compression therapy** is difficult to use on a permanent basis, another alternative for thousands of years has been **vein stripping**. In this surgical technique, the vein is detached from its insertion to the deep system near the groin and then it is pulled out of the leg down to the level of the ankle and discarded. Obviously it prevents any reflux from moving down it since the vein is removed and it relieves the subcutaneous venous hypertension which was the cause of the problems.

Vein stripping has also been used for the lesser saphenous system, which runs behind the knee down to the ankle. The operation is obviously 100% successful in relieving saphenous vein reflux since the vein is removed. Complications, however, are not insignificant and include nerve damage to the subcutaneous nerves, particularly the saphenous nerves, as well as significant pain, discoloration, and sometimes infectious morbidity. Additionally, if deep venous insufficiency is present, then this only partially solves the problem, and the patient will still have to commit to wearing extrinsic compression stockings.

Is there anything more modern, with fewer side effects?
In order to prevent the morbidity associated with vein stripping, two new techniques have been developed over the last 10 to 15 years, both of which use *endovascular technology* to ablate the vein. In this technique, a catheter is placed into the vein in the lower leg and is manipulated up the vein to the level of the groin. Then, using local anesthetic, one form of energy or another is used to destroy the vein internally, causing it to shut off its blood supply and hence end the reflux and subsequent venous hypertension. Both *laser* energy and *radio*

frequency ablation energy have been used with success, and currently the results are equal to surgery without the morbidity associated with it. It is critical for the practitioner and the patient to understand, however, that low morbidity is not the same as zero. Side effects such as *deep venous thrombosis*, *burn injury*, *nerve injury*, and recurrent or failed *recanalized veins* are a possibility and should be thoughtfully considered prior to undergoing any operation.

In summary, chronic venous insufficiency is well-known and has been documented since the earliest records of medicine 2500 years ago. The underlying problem is the loss of the ability of the veins to effectively carry blood back to the heart, resulting in blood pooling in those veins and subsequently causing fluid retention and blood retention in the subcutaneous tissues. This in turn leads to swelling and fibrosis of the subcutaneous tissue subsequently then damaging the skin and resulting in a permanent skin breakdown, pain, and disfigurement. Because all patients live in a 1G environment and cannot possibly escape the forces of gravity, the only options include counter pressure with stockings, or removal of the vein when appropriate. Scrupulous attention to risk factor modification and early intervention will almost assure an optimal outcome.

Chapter 10

Associated Diseases with PAD: Secondary Hypertension
Michael J. Gimbel, III, M.D.

Introduction
Hypertension is a disease that is frequently associated with peripheral and coronary artery disease. In the case of **peripheral arterial disease (PAD)**, hypertension can be caused or worsened by PAD. This chapter is meant to be an overview of this and other causes of **secondary hypertension**.

What is Hypertension?
Hypertension is basically the elevation of the **blood pressure** measurement (usually referred to by patients as **high blood pressure**). By definition, this elevation is a systolic blood pressure above 140 mmHg or a diastolic blood pressure above 90 mmHg. This is commonly reported as a blood pressure of 140/90 mmHg (stated 140 over 90). This should be measured at least twice on the initial evaluation, as one's blood pressure varies with **stress**, **exercise** and many other variables. This should also be repeated on follow-up visits. Measurements throughout the day during usual activities may also be helpful. **Optimal blood pressure** is less than 120/80 mmHg. Blood pressures

95

above 120/80 mmHg expose increasing risk of complications. This risk must be weighed against the risk of adverse events with treatment. Unusually **low blood pressures** may also need to be investigated, but will not be addressed here.

How common is Hypertension?
Hypertension is very common in the United States. The **American College of Cardiology (ACC)** states that about 1 in 4 adult Americans has hypertension, and that many of these are unaware of it. The frequency of hypertension increases as the population ages; with those above 80 years of age, about 60% have hypertension.

Why are we concerned about Hypertension?
The **American Heart Association (AHA)** published a report in 2003 that places the direct and indirect costs of hypertension at more than $50 billion annually. The cost alone is very alarming, but the cause of concern for us should be that hypertension that is untreated increases the risk of **coronary artery disease** and **heart attack**, **stroke**, **kidney failure** and **peripheral arterial disease**. Treating hypertension reduces this risk. As noted above, many Americans are unaware of their hypertension. If someone does not realize that he or she has hypertension, then it cannot be treated.

What is the goal of treating Hypertension?
The overall goal is to decrease the complications

of hypertension, like stroke and heart attack. The goal for most people is to have their blood pressure less than 140/90 mmHg. However, there are some people that should have their blood pressures even lower. People with **diabetes** should have their blood pressure goal less than 130/85 mmHg. Those with diabetes, **renal insufficiency** and **leakage of protein in** their **urine** should have their goal less than 125/75 mmHg. If someone has coronary artery disease and **chest pain**, their goal may also be more aggressive. Those with **congestive heart failure** may also have a lower goal for their blood pressure, but that is because the lower blood pressure may help the heart pump better, not for reducing complications of hypertension.

Is there anything I can do to help prevent or treat Hypertension, other than medications?
Non-pharmacologic therapy of hypertension includes **exercise**, **avoidance of nicotine**, **weight control**, limiting **sodium** intake, **alcohol** intake and **caffeine** intake. The most common treatment for hypertension is with **medications**. Most of the time the medication or medications can be taken only once or twice a day. Many of these medications are generic and are relatively inexpensive. If you are having trouble paying for your medications, please discuss this with your physician as there are choices in medications and some programs that may help you with your medications. **Do not just stop your medications without speaking with your doctor.**

Are there any symptoms of Hypertension?

There are usually no **symptoms** for people with moderate hypertension in the short-term. Occasionally, someone with severe hypertension, say >180mmHg systolic, may have a **headache**, **dizziness**, **chest pain**, **visual changes** or other **neurologic symptoms**. If this is the case, then urgent evaluation is needed immediately. The problem with hypertension is that people usually do not feel bad with it until its complications are manifest. This is why it is very important for screening blood pressure monitoring with your doctor, so that there can be an intervention prior to any complications occurring.

What is the usual treatment of Essential (Primary) Hypertension?

As briefly mentioned above, the treatment of hypertension is primarily a treatment consisting of medications. Exercise, reduction in caffeine and alcohol intake, weight reduction and limiting sodium intake may also be helpful. The choice of medication should be left to you and your physician as certain other conditions (like diabetes) may influence the decision of which anti-hypertensive medication may be best for you (**ACE-Inhibitor** or **ARB** for diabetics). Most of these medications are very safe and well- tolerated, but each has a side-effect profile that should be discussed. It is not uncommon that more than one medication is needed to adequately control the blood pressure and this should not be discouraging to the physician or the patient.

98

What is Secondary Hypertension?

Secondary hypertension is hypertension that is caused by an identifiable source. This is important because some causes of secondary hypertension are treated with surgery or specific medical therapy.

How common is Secondary Hypertension?

Secondary hypertension is actually not very common in the scope of hypertensive patients. The vast majority (>90%) of people with hypertension have Essential, or Primary, Hypertension. These patients have no identifiable cause for their high blood pressure.

When should Secondary Hypertension be suspected?

There are certain **"red flags"** that many clinicians look for when evaluating a patient with hypertension. One is the **severity** of the hypertension. If someone has severely elevated blood pressures, say >180/110 mmHg. Another is the **age of onset**. If the person has the onset of hypertension when they are <20 years or >50 years old, then further evaluation may be considered. If the person is not responding well to usual medical therapy, there may be another reason for his or her high blood pressure. There are also **physical exam findings** and simple **lab findings** that may be concerning. If there is evidence of **end-organ damage** (complications from the high blood pressure when diagnosed), then secondary hypertension is more prevalent. These include **retinal damage**, **elevated creatinine** (measurement of renal function),

99

and evidence of an **enlarged heart** on chest X-ray or EKG. **Low potassium**, **abdominal bruit** (swooshing sound in the abdomen on exam), **high heart rate**, **tremor** and **sweating** may also lower the threshold for further testing.

What are the causes of Secondary Hypertension?

There is a laundry list of causes of secondary hypertension.   The general causes can be broken down into groups. These include problems with the kidneys themselves, **vascular problems** with getting blood flow to the kidneys, **hormonal problems** (including **tumors** and **ingested hormones**), **neurologic problems**, **pregnancy** (**pre-eclampsia** or **eclampsia**), acute **stress** (**surgery**, **illness**) and **drug ingestion**. As stated above, many of these can be adequately evaluated with a routine history and physical by your doctor. Some of these require more testing, which will be discussed below.

What is Renovascular Hypertension and why is it important in peripheral vascular disease?

Renovascular hypertension is hypertension that is caused by reduced blood flow to the **kidneys**. This may be one kidney (unilateral) or both kidneys (bilateral). I also would include **aortic obstruction** that is above the renal arteries because the mechanism is the same. This includes **coarctation of the aorta** in this group. As this is a separate disease, this will be discussed in the next section. The reason it is

100

important in peripheral vascular disease patients is that they co-exist quite frequently.

In about 25% of patients with peripheral vascular disease, there is evidence of significant **renal artery stenosis**. Also, about 5-7% of patients over age 65 have renal artery stenosis. There are two main reasons that the arteries leading to the kidneys may become obstructed. These are **atherosclerotic disease** and **fibromuscular dysplasia**. These diseases occur in different patient populations in that fibromuscular dysplasia usually impacts younger women (less than 30 years old), whereas atherosclerotic disease impacts an older group. Fibromuscular dysplasias may impact the entire length of the renal arteries and atherosclerotic stenoses usually affect the first 1/3 of the artery. This obstruction of flow to the kidney(s) makes the kidney think that the blood pressure is low, when it is actually high. It is like a hose that is going full blast, but someone steps on the hose, causing the water to only trickle out. The kidney responds by increasing hormone (primarily renin) levels and retaining fluid to increase the blood pressure. They can both be screened for by **ultrasound** evaluation, **CT angiography**, **nuclear medicine** study or invasive **angiography**. I would not usually include an invasive test (angiography) in a group of screening tests, but in the above study, 27% of patients with lower extremity vascular disease had renal artery stenosis on angiography.

Treatment of renovascular hypertension consists

of medical therapy and invasive therapy. Invasive therapy usually consists of angioplasty and/or **stenting**, but may include surgery. Angioplasty alone is usually helpful for those with fibromuscular dysplasia whose stenoses are amenable to this. Angioplasty and stenting, if needed, also seems to help those with atherosclerotic disease.

Now, it is not very common that these interventions would cure the hypertension, as some renal damage may have occurred and there may be underlying essential hypertension, but it may reduce the number of medications needed to control the blood pressure and may decrease the decline in renal function that often occurs. There is currently considerable debate on the usefulness of revascularization in people without acute renal insufficiency or heart failures. Decisions on the therapy should be made by the patient and his or her doctor.

What about all of the other causes of Secondary Hypertension?

Secondary hypertension is pretty rare, <10% of those with hypertension. In patients with peripheral vascular disease, about ¼ of them have evidence of renal artery stenosis. This leaves a litany of problems causing <8% of the rest. As stated above, they can be arranged in some order, so they will be addressed in generalities and the most common of the rare disorders discussed.

102

What is Coarctation of the Aorta?

Coarctation of the aorta is a congenital anomaly in that there is a narrowing of the aorta, usually at the arch, that causes obstruction of flow. This is most commonly found prior to the left *subclavian artery*, so the blood pressure in the right arm is usually higher than that found in the left. The result of the stenosis is decreased blood flow to the left arm and the lower body. As the kidneys see less blood flow, they respond by producing hormones to increase the blood pressure. This is suspected by differential blood pressures in the arms, rib notching on chest X-ray, and occasionally symptoms of left arm pain with use and lower extremity *claudication*. This should also be suspected in a younger patient as it can be present from birth. This is addressed either surgically or, more recently, percuataneous options have been performed.

What causes kidney disease and hypertension?

As stated above, renovascular disease causes hypertension. *Intrinsic kidney disease* also causes it. This can be in an acute setting or chronic. These include many diseases, including *diabetic nephropathy*, *glomerulonephritis*, *vasculitis*, *pyelonephritis*, *analgesic nephropathy* and many others. The treatment of these is to medically control the blood pressure and treat the underlying renal problem, if possible. *ACE-Inhibitors* and *Angiotensin Receptor Blockers* are beneficial in patients with diabetic nephropathy, if they can take them.

Can hormonal problems cause hypertension?

Yes, they can. This may be from normal tissues gone awry, ingested hormones or from tumor-producing hormones. The **adrenal glands** normally produce hormones, but benign **adenomas** can produce them in levels too high. There are also **congenital problems** that can cause hypertension, but these are usually found in children. A malignant tumor called a **pheochromocytoma** can also produce hormones that cause hypertension. They are usually in the adrenal gland, but may be elsewhere. The treatment for adrenal adenomas and pheochromocytoma is removal, if possible. A particular medication called an **alpha blocker** is particularly useful in combination with a **beta blocker**. Another hormone that can cause hypertension is **Serotonin**. **Carcinoid tumors** can cause hypertension and the treatment targets the tumors. **Low thyroid hormone levels**, **high parathyroid hormone** and **high growth hormone levels** can also cause hypertension. These are treated by correcting the hormonal problem. **Exogenous steroids** and **growth hormone** can also cause hypertension. The last hormonal problem to be discussed is hypertension with oral contraceptive use. This is usually mild, but may persist after discontinuation.

What is Obstructive Sleep Apnea?

Obstructive sleep apnea is a condition where, as a person is sleeping, their airway is occasionally obstructed. This causes the

104

body to work harder to try to get air in and increases sympathetic activity. This is the same mechanism of the *"fight or flight response"* where your heart rate increases, blood pressure increases and you get ready for confrontation. This all occurs while they are still asleep, but the sleep is restless. Sometimes people have *fatigue*, fall asleep easily, headache in the morning and usually report *snoring* (by a relative or spouse). An overnight test in the hospital is usually required for evaluation and this can usually be treated with a special mask worn at night to keep the airway from closing. Occasionally, surgery may be needed. This treatment reduces the sympathetic activity and improves the symptoms and blood pressure control. This is important because it is easily diagnosed if it is diagnosed and can be treated effectively.

What is the "usual" work-up for possible Secondary Hypertension?

This is usually targeted by the patient and the findings on preliminary tests. The initial lab work-up usually consists of *blood tests* for blood counts, kidney, thyroid, liver and electrolyte levels. An *EKG* is almost always done for both a baseline and to evaluate for *left ventricular hypertrophy*. If there is concern for renal artery stenosis, then an ultrasound evaluation of the kidneys and renal arteries is usually sufficient for initial evaluation. A 24-hour urine collection for metanephrines (to evaluate for pheochromocytoma), 5-HIAA (to evaluate for carcinoid syndrome) and potassium (if the serum potassium is low, to evaluate for primary hyperaldosteronism) may be performed. Further imaging (CT scan or MRI) may be done if these are abnormal. Much of the work-up is contingent on the initial tests, index of suspicion and the manifestation of the hypertension.

Conclusion
Hypertension is extremely common in patients with peripheral vascular disease. The majority of the time, it is likely to be essential hypertension. It is not uncommon for these patients to have secondary hypertension, or have another cause. This should be suspected if there is an acute change, severe hypertension, poor response to therapy or other exam findings. Of the causes of secondary hypertension in this patient population, renovascular hypertension is the most common. This can be assessed non-invasively easily. There is debate about the utility of angioplasty and stenting, but this should be discussed with the patient and doctor. There are other, treatable problems that can cause hypertension. These include hormonal, congenital, malignant and exogenous causes. These can be evaluated and treated with blood tests, imaging and a good physical exam and history. Treatment of hypertension reduces the long term risk of cardiovascular complications. Hypertension is usually asymptomatic, so evaluation with periodic blood pressure measurements is needed to avoid these complications.

Chapter 11

How Heart Disease can be Affected by Peripheral Artery Disease
Nicolas W. Shammas, MD, MS

What is the relationship between heart disease and PAD?
The blood vessels of the heart, legs and brain are all part of the same vascular system and are affected by the same type of *plaque build-up*. It is not uncommon to find patients with *PAD* who also have blockages in their heart arteries (*coronaries*) and the arteries of their brain (*carotids*). Patients with PAD are at an exceptionally high risk for heart attacks and strokes. In one study, patients over the age of 50 with PAD had a 68% and 42% incidence of coexistent coronary artery disease and stroke respectively. Also, the more symptomatic the PAD, the more likely a patient will die of heart disease or stroke rather than from the complications of PAD itself. Mortality due to heart disease was 15-fold more among symptomatic subjects with severe large-vessel PAD. Finally, PAD has been classified as a coronary artery risk equivalent, i.e., carrying

more than 20% risk of a coronary event in 10 years.

In this chapter, the focus will be on heart disease and the impact of blockages in the coronaries. This chapter is a slight modification from the one published in the prior book of our Foundation "Learn about Your Heart Made Simple" (edited by Shammas NW).

How does the heart receive its blood supply?

The heart is a pump that continuously beats at 60 to 100 beats per minute during the life of a person. This pump requires oxygen and nutrients to achieve its tasks. These are delivered to the heart via **blood vessels** called the **coronaries**. There are three or four major **coronary arteries** that deliver blood to the heart. These supply the top (left anterior descending artery), the side (the left circumflex), and the bottom (the right coronary artery) of the heart. Any interruption of blood supply to any of those coronaries can lead to heart damage to a correspondent part of the heart muscle.

How do the coronaries fill up with plaque and become obstructed?

The coronaries are covered on the inside by a lining called the **endothelium**, a single layer of cells that covers every single blood vessel in our body. It has been estimated that if this lining of all the blood vessels from one individual is spread on a flat surface, it could cover two

108

tennis courts in size. This single layer of cells, however, separates the blood vessels from health and disease.

Any damage to the endothelium can lead to its invasion by blood elements called **monocytes**. These monocytes penetrate under the lining of those blood vessels and absorb fat from the bloodstream. They become enlarged in size and are called **foam cells**. These foam cells promote a complex reaction under the endothelium, which subsequently causes **inflammation** and attracts various other cells to the plaque area. The plaque expands and starts to impinge on the opening of the blood vessels that supply the heart.

It is well known that the process of **plaque formation** starts very early in childhood. Autopsies on young soldiers who died in wars have shown that the blood vessels of their bodies already show the build-up of fat under the endothelium. Over two-thirds of people over the age of 40 show the build up of plaque in the blood vessels that supply their heart, as seen by ultrasound scanning of those blood vessels.

What is angina?
Angina is a symptom of **chest pain** – also described as **chest pressure**, a heavy feeling in the chest, a squeezing sensation in the chest – which is caused by a lack of blood supply to a part of the heart muscle. Angina is described as either stable or unstable.

A narrowing in one of the blood vessels of the heart by plaque build-up causes **stable angina**. Stable angina occurs when a person is active and doing physical exertion. It typically resolves within two to three minutes of resting. This type of angina does not occur at rest. As a person becomes active and exerts himself or herself, the heart has to pump faster and stronger. With the increase in the heart rate, there is a need to increase the blood supply to the heart to continue to match its demands. If plaque build-up is severe enough to narrow the coronaries, then the blood supply to the heart cannot increase at the rate needed by the heart. A mismatch of demand and blood supply occurs. This generates discomfort in the heart – angina. Once the patient rests and the demands of the heart for blood supply returns to normal, then the pain resolves. This process is very similar to claudication in patients with PAD. As blood supply diminishes to the leg that is exercising because of a blockage in the peripheral arteries, then acid accumulates in the leg and a cramping painful sensation occurs in the calf muscle. With few minutes of rest this resolves and a patient is able to walk again until the same type of pain recurs again.

In contrast to stable angina, a rupture of the plaque inside the blood vessels causes **unstable angina**. This leads to a subsequent accumulation of a clot at the area of the plaque rupture, which abruptly interrupts the blood supply to the heart. Angina then occurs with very minimal activity or at rest. *This type of angina requires immediate medical attention.*

This is also very similar to what could happen with some PAD patient where a sudden clot forms in the arteries of the leg interrupting the blood supply to the lower extremity. This could lead to **gangrene** or **tissue death** if not addressed on an emergency basis and treated. Patients with PAD should present themselves to the emergency room when a sudden, unexplained pain occurs in their lower foot with a change in the color of the foot or alteration of the sensation in the foot.

How does the patient perceive angina?
Angina is perceived as chest pressure, tightness, a squeeze, or heaviness in the chest. This could radiate to the arm and the jaw, the shoulders, the back, or the abdomen. The pain can be associated with an increase in shortness of breath, a feeling of nausea, and occasional vomiting. Also, patients break out in a sweat, which we call **diaphoresis**. **Lightheadedness** and **anxiety** accompany those symptoms. Patients might describe one or more of these symptoms, on many occasions, without any chest discomfort. Females and diabetics tend to present with atypical symptoms without chest pain. In the legs, **claudication** is also perceived as a pain sensation in the calf muscle that resolves with rest. It can radiate to the thigh or the foot.

What should you do if you experience chest pain or other symptoms of angina?
If you experience chest pain or any of the symptoms described above, is important that you not attempt to self-diagnose. *It is very important in this situation to seek immediate medical attention.* If the pain occurs at rest, this is essentially an emergency, and driving to the hospital or having someone to drive you can be very dangerous. The best way to deal with your *rest angina* is to call 9-1-1 and allow paramedics to transport you to the hospital. The first hour of the onset of the chest discomfort is the most dangerous. Electrical disturbances in the heart can occur and the heart could cease pumping blood to the brain and the vital organs of the body. This can be easily corrected if you are being transported to the hospital with trained professionals. However, *sudden cardiac death* can occur if you are still at home or you are in a regular car on your way to the hospital. A sudden change in symptoms – such as the occurrence of nausea or vomiting, sudden worsening of breathing, or the occurrence of chest pain – all warrant immediate hospital evaluation.

If the chest pain or the anginal symptoms have been occurring primarily with exertion or activity, but never at rest, this tends to be somewhat less of an emergency. However, evaluation should be performed relatively soon. Calling your doctor and getting evaluated relatively soon is important. The symptoms of *pain with exertion* are classic anginal

112

symptoms and they have a high chance to be related to obstructive plaque in the coronary arteries.

Claudication, or pain with exertion in the lower extremity, is typically not an emergency, and a person can drive his or her car to the doctor's office to be checked on a routine basis. However, sudden rest pain in the leg is an emergency and a patient can present to the emergency room driven by ambulance or by a friend/relative. However, presenting to the emergency room should be quick if the symptoms occur at rest and were sudden in nature.

How does a patient die from a heart attack?
The most common cause of death from *heart attack* is electrical instability to the heart. Once the blood supply is interrupted, the electrical conduction inside the heart becomes disturbed. Abnormal electrical circuits are generated in the bottom chambers of the heart. These lead to quivering of the heart muscle. The heart muscle becomes very inefficient in pumping blood. These arrhythmias are called *ventricular tachycardia* or *ventricular fibrillation*. The blood will be able to generate minimal to no blood supply to the vital organs of the body, including the brain. A person loses consciousness usually within 5 to 10 seconds of the occurrence of this event. Death occurs if the electrical system of the heart is not restored back to its normal condition within 5 to 6 minutes of the electrical disturbance. Rarely, heart failure resulting from the heart

attack leads to death. By far, the majority of deaths are related to this electrical instability. Paramedics and hospitals are equipped with machines called **defibrillators** that are capable of aborting those electrical heart rhythms by delivering an electrical shock to the chest. Automatic external defibrillators are now widely placed in public places such as airports, schools, and large business centers. **Operation Heartbeat**, a program of the **American Heart Association**, has intended to extend the use of automatic external defibrillators in public places in order to save lives of heart attack victims.

Cardiopulmonary resuscitation, which includes artificial respiration and chest compression, can sustain enough of a blood circulation for the first 10 minutes after the electrical instability has occurred.

However, without the more definitive therapy of defibrillation using the defibrillator, cardiopulmonary resuscitation is inadequate alone to restore a normal heart rhythm. In fact, survival rate after six minutes of the arrhythmia is slim despite cardiopulmonary resuscitation and without defibrillation.

What does my doctor do when I come to the emergency room with chest pain?
Your doctor will evaluate you with a full history and physical exam. Details of the chest pain such as its onset, severity, radiation, and association with other symptoms or with activity will all be important information to provide. A

114

physical exam to listen to your lungs and heart will be important. Based on all the information gathered, including blood testing, your physician will attempt to determine whether your symptoms could be related to your heart or are noncardiac in origin.

If it is a possibility that these symptoms are heart-related, then you will be asked to stay in the hospital. Many hospitals have a chest pain unit where you will be observed for several hours on a monitor. **Serial blood testing** will be obtained to rule out the possibility of heart injury. An **electrocardiogram** also will be obtained. Eventually, if all your tests are unremarkable, a stress test will be performed.

All these tests will help your doctor to decide whether to admit you to the hospital for further workup, such as a **coronary angiogram**. On the other hand, if your chest pain has occurred at rest and continues to do so in the emergency room, your doctor will have to assume that this is an unstable anginal symptom. You will then be directly admitted to the hospital and placed on medical treatment. If the suspicion for cardiac-related symptoms is high, then your doctor might proceed directly with an angiogram.

What is a cardiac catheterization or a coronary angiogram?
A **cardiac catheterization** is essentially the same as a **coronary angiogram**. This procedure is performed in the cardiac

catheterization laboratory. During this procedure, a small plastic tube is inserted in the blood vessels in the groin, called the **common femoral artery**. This small plastic tube or catheter is placed under a local anesthetic. Through this catheter, plastic tubes are placed inside the blood vessels under x-ray guidance. These go to the heart, where a contrast dye is injected. The dye is injected directly in the heart's chamber as well as in the blood vessels of your heart. As the dye is being injected in those blood vessels, a camera takes multiple pictures of your heart, which will allow your physician to see your coronaries and determine the location of the blockages, if present.

The angiogram is considered an invasive procedure. It does carry some risks with it. These risks vary depending on the condition of the patient. Patients with heart failure and reduced heart function, diabetes or kidney problems tend to be at exceptionally high risk. Patients with previous history of heart attacks, strokes, and blockages in the blood vessels of the legs are also at higher risk. However, the overall risks of the procedure remain small. In a non-emergent angiogram, the risk of death should be less than 1 in a 1000, risk of strokes 1 in 500, and the risk of major bleeding from the insertion site of the catheter should be less than 1%. Obviously, these risks also vary if the angiogram is only for diagnostic purposes to identify the location of the blockage or for treatment purposes to treat the blockage.

During the treatment of blockages, large amounts of **blood thinners** are administered, which increases the risk of bleeding and complications. Other risks of the angiogram also include infection, damage to the nerves in the groin area, damage to the arteries of the heart themselves, as well as the aorta, the main artery that comes out of the heart and supplies blood to the rest of the body. Your doctor will weigh carefully all those risks compared to the potential benefits of the test.

Typically, an **informed consent** – a legal contract that authorizes the physician to proceed with the test – is obtained after you understand these risks and your questions and concerns are answered. Signing a **consent form** essentially acknowledges your understanding to these risks and your willingness to proceed with the test. You should treat it seriously, carefully read it, and understand it. The physician or the nurse should be available to answer any questions you might have.

How do we treat blockages in the coronaries once they are found?

Blockages in the blood vessels of the heart are treated in three different ways.

1) Your doctor might decide that your coronary blockages are only borderline in nature or insignificant and preventative therapy and medical therapy might be advised.

2) If your blockages, however, are severe, then the treatment can be done by either an **angioplasty** or a **bypass surgery**. During an

angioplasty, your cardiologist passes a balloon into the blocked arteries. Once the balloon is inflated at the area of the blockage *(see picture)*, the blockage will be compressed and the artery is stretched. A **stent**, or a stainless steel mesh, is most frequently deployed in the area of the treatment to keep the artery widely open and prevent it from collapse. The choice of the stent depends on the type of blockages, their location, and the ability to deliver the stent to that part of your coronaries.

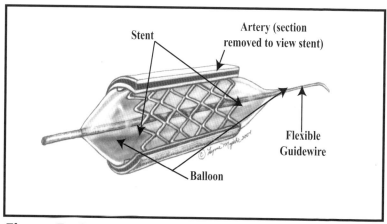

Figure 7. *Stent mounted on balloon in artery*

Although the current standard of treating blockages is with the use of a stent, some blockages are not amenable to stenting because of their size or the difficulty of delivering the stents to a particular blockage because of blood vessel **tortuosity** and **calcification**. Current stents also have medications in them. These medications prevent the recurrence of blockages within the area of the treatment. The choice

118

of the stents is also guided by certain rules that your doctor might follow. Currently, the majority of the blockages are managed through the angioplasty process.

3) However, some blockages might be in locations too dangerous to treat with angioplasty or might be extensive for an angioplasty procedure. They might be complex in nature and particularly if this occurs in a diabetic. Currently, the trend is to treat those blockages with the **bypass operation**. During the bypass operation, a blood vessel under the collarbone and/or a vein derived from under the skin of the legs is utilized to bypass the area of the blockage.

How long does it take to recover from the treatment of a blockage in the heart?
If an angioplasty is utilized as the primary method of treating a blockage, then generally you stay in the hospital for 23 hours. Within 72 hours, you should be able to drive and resume your normal activities.

The exception to this is if you have had a heart attack. After a heart attack, typically a patient cannot drive for two weeks and should be undergoing cardiac rehabilitation for a minimum of four weeks prior to **release back to work**. Your doctor will decide on the size of heart attack that you had, the extent of cardiac rehabilitation required, and the optimal time for you to return to work.

On the other hand, bypass surgery would require that you stay in the hospital for an average of four to five days. This can be significantly more prolonged if complications would occur. The recovery phase is in the range of about six weeks. For about three months, you should avoid carrying any weight that exceeds 10 pounds, avoiding any form of exertion that would require pulling and pushing. It is also important to minimize any trauma to the area of the wound in the middle of the chest. Driving typically is not permitted during the first month after bypass surgery.

There are many exceptions to the above rules based on your condition, complications occurring during surgery, and your recovery.

What is the long-term outcome following treatment of blockages in the heart?

Following the treatment of a blockage with an angioplasty, there is an immediate inflammation that occurs at the site of the treatment. This response of the blood vessel to the injury that the balloon has caused triggers the formation of *scar tissue* at the site of the treatment. Patients develop scar tissue to a different extent for unclear reasons. The scar tissue that develops within the stent can potentially cause a recurrence of a blockage in the area of the treatment.

When balloon angioplasty alone was utilized without stenting, the recurrence of the blockage was in the range of about 40%. When a stent

120

is used, the recurrence of a blockage is in the range of 15 to 20%.

Higher rate of recurrence occurs in diabetics, patients with small blood vessels, and those with long areas of blockages.

With the advent of the stents loaded with drugs that suppress these **blockages (drug-eluting stents)**, the rate of recurrence of scar tissue is currently about 5 to 9%.

It is typical for scar tissue to form within the first six months of an angioplasty. If this does not occur within the first six months, it is less likely that it will occur afterwards.

Your doctor might elect to proceed with a **stress test** at about four to six months following an angioplasty to determine whether enough scar tissue has occurred to block the artery again. The decision to do this stress test is generally a clinical one and physician-dependent.

The overall outcome of the patient, however, from the standpoint of preventing a heart attack is mostly dependent on preventative measures rather than the angioplasty process itself. In other words, angioplasty for blockages that has caused no symptoms or only stable symptoms generally does not affect a person's survival. The major impact of angioplasty is on improving the quality of life and lessening the need for medications.

In order to prevent death or a heart attack long-term, strict control of cardiac risk factors becomes important. This includes controlling the blood pressure, cholesterol, blood sugar, the weight, and avoiding smoking. **Dietary modification**, **exercise**, and **stress reduction** also become very important.

Following a bypass surgery, the procedure's long-term success depends on the continued normal functioning of the **bypass grafts**. It is known that 10 to 15% of bypass grafts can deteriorate within the first year of surgery. Also, at about 10 years from a bypass, two-thirds of all bypasses are expected to have significant amount of build-up of plaques and blockages. There has been a lot of progress made recently in the treatment of those bypass grafts.

However, again, the overall long-term survival and benefit is highly dependent on preventative measures. Several studies have indicated that the viability of bypass grafts and their overall health is related to taking blood thinners, such as aspirin or clopidogrel, and the use of some cholesterol-lowering medications such as the statins. Research is continually ongoing to find ways to preserve those bypasses and prevent them from deteriorating or blocking shortly after the surgery.

What is a heart attack and how does it happen?

Heart attack happens when there is a sudden interruption of the blood supply to a part of the heart muscle. This leads to death of the muscle tissue. A heart attack leads to symptoms similar to **angina**. However, these symptoms tend to be more prolonged and generally are more than a half-hour in duration. The interruption of the blood supply to the heart occurs because of a **plaque rupture**. A plaque, irrespective of severity, can break, exposing the inside of the plaque to the blood elements. The blood forms a **clot** on the top of the ruptured plaque. If the clot does not block the artery entirely, **unstable angina** certainly will occur, as described in previous questions. However, if the interruption in the blood supply is complete because of a full clot, then the muscle of the heart supplied by this particular blood vessel will be deprived of nutrients and oxygen and will die.

The most important step in the management of a heart attack is to restore the blood supply to the heart muscle as quickly as possible. The current guidelines strongly suggest that the artery should be opened with the **angioplasty** procedure within 90 minutes of a patient's arrival to the emergency room. If the angioplasty procedure is not available to this particular emergency room and hospital, then the use of a clot-dissolving (or **thrombolytic**) medicine needs to be used immediately, within 30 minutes of arrival to the emergency room. Most hospitals are able to initiate the use of these thrombolytic drugs within about 20 minutes of a patient arriving to the emergency room.

Current data strongly suggest, however, that the angioplasty is a more effective way of opening up an artery in a heart attack situation, and probably leads to a better short- and long-term outcome.

Therefore, it is imperative that when the pain starts or when symptoms of a heart attack start, the patient needs to be **transported to an emergency room** as soon as possible. Time is extremely precious, and the longer the delay in opening a closed artery, the more damage will happen to the heart muscle. In fact, in four to six hours after the artery is closed, the damage is essentially complete. There is strong data to suggest that the earlier the artery is opened, the higher the likelihood of survival from a heart attack.

What medications should I expect to be taking following a heart attack?

Following the acute treatment of a heart attack, which is primarily restoring the blood supply to the heart muscle, a patient is placed on several medications to reduce the chance of another heart attack and and therefore reduce the likelihood of death

The standard therapy consists of the use of a **beta-blocker** that has been shown to reduce heart failure, arrhythmias, and prevent stretching and dilatation of the heart muscle following a heart attack.

In addition, the patient is expected to be

124

on a *statin*, which is a cholesterol-lowering medication that has also shown to substantially prevent the chance of another heart attack. The use of *blood thinners* such as *aspirin* and *clopidogrel (Plavix)* has become standard therapy to also reduce the chance of another cardiac event. The use of an *angiotensin-converting enzyme (ACE) inhibitor* in patients following a heart attack and reduced left ventricular function is also now a standard to prolong life and reduce the chance of further cardiovascular events.

With the use of a **beta-blocker**, an *ACE inhibitor*, *aspirin*, *clopidogrel*, and a *statin*, one would expect that the *chance of recurrence of a heart attack* should be reduced to less than 3% per year on this preventative therapy.

In addition to *pharmacologic therapy*, the patient will be strongly advised to watch strict *dietary restrictions*, *weight control*, *exercise*, and adhering to a *no-smoking policy*. All these changes require significant *lifestyle modifications*, which at times can be challenging. However, a patient striving for better health generally has strong motivation to follow these guidelines to prevent another heart attack.

How important is Cardiac Rehabilitation after a heart attack or a bypass surgery?
Cardiac Rehabilitation in a structured format, with the patient being monitored, has been

shown to substantially improve the quality of life, with data also suggesting an improvement in survival. Cardiac Rehabilitation allows patients to gain confidence in their ability to do things, gradually increases their fitness level, and helps them develop a habit to exercise routinely on a long-term basis.

The importance of exercise is mostly in its **cardiovascular fitness** and **conditioning** that allows a stronger ability of the body to extract **oxygen** from the blood, as well as improve the overall efficiency of the heart. A trained and fit individual tends to have a slower heart rate at rest and a lower **adrenaline** blood level. These are very protective elements overall to the heart.

Cardiac Rehabilitation is very strongly recommended to cardiac patients after an angioplasty, a heart attack, or bypass surgery. Many patients see a tremendous improvement in their sense of well-being and an improvement in their depression after a heart attack. This, in itself, also has significant protective effect to their overall health as well as cardiovascular health.

The second phase of Cardiac Rehabilitation is the **outpatient** phase that follows a heart attack and is generally monitored under the guidance of cardiac rehabilitation nurses or technicians. The patient is generally placed on a monitor and different kinds of exercises are encouraged, with close monitoring of the heart rates and the blood

126

pressure, as well as the heart rhythm. A gradual increase in the **target heart rate** is done under the guidance of the primary cardiologist.

The third phase of Cardiac Rehabilitation is a less-monitored phase where a person joins a group of heart patients and exercises on a routine basis. Phase III provides significant group support to the heart patient and allows uninterrupted, continued exercise with minimal supervision, but with some sort of ongoing guidance.

Chapter 12

Diseases of the Aorta: Aortic Dissections versus Aneurysms
Richard Sadler, MD, FACS

Many patients inquire about *aortic aneurysms* and the risks associated with them, especially since screening tests are now available and reimbursed by some insurance carriers.

However, although aneurysms are a potential threat, they actually are **not** the biggest threat to patients. The #1 killer is a lesser-known but much more common malady called an *aortic dissection*.

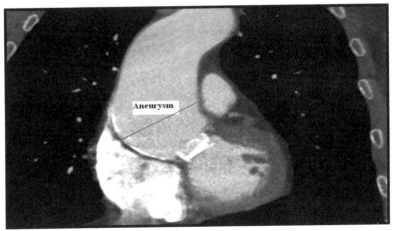

Figure 8. *Ascending aortic aneurysm*

How often do aortic dissections occur?

Aortic dissection is the most common catastrophe of the **aorta**, 2 to 3 times more common than rupture of the abdominal aorta. When left untreated, about 50% of patients die within the first 24 hours, and 60% die within 48 hours. The 2-week mortality rate approaches 90% in patients with undiagnosed ascending aortic dissection (the portion of the aorta that arises from the heart). In short, 1-2% of patients die every hour from the time it starts!

The dissections within the first 20 cm or 7 inches of the aorta (called Type A) are the most lethal, with 90% of patients dying within the first week without treatment. If complications occur, death may be inevitable. Those that occur further away from the heart, in the descending aorta (type B) are less dangerous, but can still be fatal without some form of treatment.

What exactly is a dissection?

The essential feature of aortic dissection is a tear in the intimal (or inside) layer, followed by formation and propagation of a **subintimal hematoma** (a collection of blood under the inner lining of the aorta). The blood within the aorta actually splits the vessel wall, moving both forward and backward, causing bleeding, shearing off other vessels to vital organs and causing bleeding around the heart, which is usually fatal. This is called a **tamponade** and is a critical event.

How do patients feel and how do they know they have it?

First, it is absolutely critical to understand that even though a patient may have risk factors, a dissection is not a slow, progressive disease like an aneurysm. The patient's aorta is intact and essentially normal until the split occurs. There is NO screening test, because the disease does not exist until the tear! Patients can only know they have an aortic dissection when the signs and symptoms start.

Are the signs and symptoms easy to feel or unique to dissections?

NO! Although there is no mistaking that the patient has strong symptoms and clearly feels ill, the symptoms are what we call protean, meaning that it may feel many different ways and feel like many other diseases. This tendency to act like other diseases is what makes aortic dissections so treacherous!

Is there a special pattern to look for?

Yes, and this pattern is critical to making the diagnosis.

The pain usually is described as **ripping** or **tearing**. The description of ripping or tearing has been shown to increase the chance that an aortic dissection has occurred. The sudden onset of chest pain has been shown to occur in 84% of patients with aortic dissection.

However, this description is not universal, and some patients present with only mild pain, often mistaken for musculoskeletal conditions, located in the thorax, groin, or back.

The pain of aortic dissection typically is distinguished from the pain of a heart attack by its abrupt onset.

Aortic dissection should be considered strongly in all patients reporting acute, sudden, and severe chest pain that is maximal at onset.

There is one presentation that is almost diagnostic however, and that is the presence of "migrating chest pain." This means that the pain may start in the chest, then move in a sequential manner to the neck, shoulders, back, flank, then abdomen, representing the progressive tearing seen in the natural history of dissections.

Do all patients have chest pain?
NO! Other presentations include:

- *Neurologic symptoms*
- *Syncope* (fainting)
- *Stroke symptoms* (Weak arm or leg; altered sensation)
- *Altered mental status*
- *Limb tingling* and *numbness*, *pain*, or *weakness*
- *Hemiparesis* or *hemiplegia* (*paralysis*)
- *Horner syndrome* (a droopy face and dilated pupil)

Other non specific symptoms include:

132

- *Dyspnea* (difficulty breathing)
- *Dysphagia* (difficulty swallowing)
- *Orthopnea* (difficultly breathing when lying down)
- *Anxiety* and *premonitions of death*
- *Flank pain* if the artery of the kidney is involved
- *Dyspnea* and *hemoptysis* (coughing blood) if dissection ruptures into the lining of the lung
- *Tachycardia* (high heart rate associated with heart compromise)
- *Shock* (low blood pressure seen with blood compressing the heart and bleeding)

What are the risk factors for getting a dissection?

It is typically having a higher blood pressure seen in conjunction with:

Hereditary diseases, such as:
- *Marfan syndrome*
- *Ehlers-Danlos syndrome*
- *Annuloaortic ectasia*
- *Familial aortic dissections*
- *Adult polycystic kidney disease*
- *Turner syndrome*
- *Noonan syndrome*
- *Osteogenesis imperfecta*
- *Bicuspid aortic valve*
- *Coarctation of the aorta*
- *Connective tissue disorders*
- *Metabolic disorders* (e.g., *homocystinuria, familial hypercholesterolemia*)

Non-hereditary diseases, including:

- In an estimated 50% of all cases of aortic dissection that occur in women younger than 40 years are associated with **pregnancy**
- **Syphilis** may cause aortic dissection
- **Crack cocaine** use may precipitate aortic dissection
- **Iatrogenic** causes of aortic dissection include **cardiac catheterization**

How does the doctor make a diagnosis?
Although physicians pay close attention to the patient's story and physical examination, those findings can be very imprecise. Furthermore, the consequences of a misdiagnosis and the implications of a correct diagnosis are so profound that **imaging** is a critical diagnostic tool. This means looking at the aorta with either **ultrasound** (**echocardiography**), **Computed Tomography** (**CT**) or **Magnetic Resonance Imaging** (**MRI**).

Transesophageal echocardiography (**TEE**) gives an ultrasound picture of the aorta obtained directly by swallowing an ultrasound-tipped small tube that images the aorta directly through the **esophagus** (or the **feeding tube**). This has greater accuracy, in the range of 97-99%, to detect aortic dissection. It is very safe and gives images of high reliability. Furthermore, when it demonstrates NO dissection, then one can be confident that aortic dissection is very unlikely. It does, however, require a skilled user and interpretation.

134

Computed tomography angiography (CTA) scanning is the diagnostic test of choice in many institutions, challenging ***angiography***, which had been the accepted diagnostic criterion standard. Accuracy is greater than 95%.

More importantly, imaging information – including the type of dissection, location of the pathologic lesion, extent of the disease, and distinguishing the true from the false opening in the aorta following the tear – can be assessed quickly and help the surgeon plan the operation. Drawbacks include the following:

- CT angiography requires the injection of iodinated contrast

- The use of contrast material may harm a patient who has impaired kidney function or an allergy to contrast media

- CT scanning provides no information on leaking in the aortic valve in the heart.

These risks are probably outweighed by the major advantage of CTA, which is the ability to make other diagnoses at the same time. Of all the tests, CTA probably yields the most information that is clinically useful.

Magnetic resonance imaging (***MRI***) has 90-95% accuracy in diagnosing aortic dissection. The most sensitive method for diagnosing aortic dissection, MRI shows the site of tear in the inner lining of the aorta, the type and extent of dissection, and presence of aortic valve leak in the heart.

Other benefits are that MRI requires no contrast

medium and no exposure to x/rays. It is the preferred modality for patients with kidney problems and those with an allergy to iodine. MRI also is the preferred tool for imaging chronic tears in the aorta and follow-up after surgical repair.

Drawbacks include the following:

- MRI is not readily available at most institutions, requiring transportation of patients in unstable condition away from the emergency room.

- MRI requires much more time to acquire images than CT scanning. This long period for obtaining images makes it prohibitive in a true emergency where time is of the essence.

- Patients with permanent pacemakers cannot undergo MRI. However, most patients with prosthetic heart valves or coronary stents can safely have an MRI.

Can this be treated with medicine, or do I have to have surgery?

Although surgery is reserved for special cases *(see below),* appropriate medication is used for all patients with aortic dissection. This is due to the very special nature of this disease. Keep in mind that left untreated, it will almost certainly get worse. Furthermore, it is a dynamic disease, meaning that there is always damage being done. This is because the tear is made worse with each beat of the heart. Since it is impossible to stop the heart from doing its necessary work, the only alternative is to alter the way in which it works.

136

The degree of tearing is really a function of how much force the heart generates moving the blood forward, and the higher this force the more the tear. So remember, **it is not just how high the blood pressure gets, but how fast it gets there!**

What kind of medicines are used?
Antihypertensives are used to reduce blood pressure. The mainstay drug is a **beta blocker**, such as **Breviblock**, which works directly to alter the pressure over time. This is usually given intravenously and requires admission to an intensive care unit for close monitoring. Other beta blockers include **Lopressor**, **Inderal** and **Labetalol**.

A second-line therapy or additional medications may include **calcium channel blockers**, such as **Nifedipine or Cardizem**. This also slows down the heart's contractions.

Remember, even more important than the absolute blood pressure is the need to slow the rate of contraction in the heart!

When is surgery indicated?
Surgery is needed when there is a threat of serious complication, like stroke, or death. The goal of surgery is to stop the tearing of the aorta and to redirect blood to its normal route, making sure the vital organs are well-perfused.

In the **descending aorta**, also known as a **Stanford B dissection**, medication is often equally effective as operation. However, if bleeding suddenly develops, or organ dysfunction like kidney failure, surgery is then indicated.

Traditionally the operation was performed under general anaesthesia through a chest incision, and a **Dacron graft** is inserted to replace the torn aorta *(see Figure 2)*. The death rate was around 5-50%, depending on how bad the dissection was and where it was.

The Type A or ascending aorta is virtually always repaired with an operation. The natural history of this disease is that medications will not stop the tearing and subsequent complications of massive brain injury and cardiac compression and arrest.

This also was fixed with a Dacron graft after first stopping the heart and cooling the brain.

Recently, a newer technology has been available that shows promise. This is called a stented graft, and uses a wire stent that is covered with a **Gore-tex** membrane and placed up through the groin into the aorta itself, then opened or deployed, covering the tear and preventing further damage, while at the same time rerouting the blood into correct natural channels.

Summary:
Aortic dissection is the #1 aortic catastrophe that kills patients. This is especially dangerous since it is a sudden event, and cannot be detected until the actual threatening tear occurs.

The clinical presentation is so varied that no one syndrome is diagnostic. However, **any sudden back or chest pain that is severe, and is characterized as ripping or tearing, must be considered a dissection until proven otherwise.**

Treatment always consists of drugs that alter the force of heart contraction, and may also include operative repair by a trained heart surgeon. After successful repair, the patient must be compliant in following the medication regimen, which includes beta blockers and blood pressure medicine. Failure to take these medicines is the #1 cause of continued problems.

Chapter 13

Modifiable Risk Factors for Peripheral Arterial Disease
Nicolas W. Shammas, MD, MS

Modifiable risk factors for PAD are many and include *smoking*, *high cholesterol levels*, *high blood pressure*, *diabetes*, *obesity*, and a *poor diet*. Although older age and male gender are risk factors to develop PAD, these are non-modifiable and will not be discussed in this chapter. Various risk factors will be discussed in details in other chapters. We offer here a review of these risk factors with a focus on dietary intervention.

Are diabetics at increased risk of PAD?
Diabetes is one of the strongest risk factor for PAD. Patients with diabetes and PAD also have higher complications from PAD, including *amputations* and *death*. Diabetics with *neuropathy* (nerve damage in their lower legs), *retinopathy* (eye damage), severe *blockages* in their legs, *obesity*, and males are at a particularly high risk for diabetic complications. *Patient education* to avoid *foot injuries* and *ulcerations* is of paramount importance to reduce amputations in the diabetics. *Diabetes control* is important to reduce the chance of small-vessel damage in the eyes, kidneys and legs. It is unclear at this time whether a very

aggressive treatment of diabetes reduces the chance of an amputation in a patient with PAD.

Can smoking damage the arteries of the legs?

Smoking is also a powerful risk factor for PAD because it damages the internal lining of the arteries that protect them from developing plaque. Also, smoking increases the chance of blood clots. Cigarette smoking has been shown to be even a more powerful risk factor to develop PAD than heart disease. Current smoking of 25 or more cigarettes per day increased the chance of PAD by 7.3 times. Also, current smokers seem to have a higher rate of complications during procedures to treat PAD such as surgery or angioplasty. In addition, smokers tend to have higher unexpected problems with clotting in their arteries following treatment which require further procedures. **Smoking cessation** is an important step to reduce symptoms of **pain in the lower legs** from PAD and cardiac complications. In fact, some authorities consider smoking cessation and **exercise** to be the two most important treatments for PAD.

Does high cholesterol affect the lower leg arteries?

High cholesterol and **fat in the blood stream** (**dyslipidemia**) are significant risk factors for PAD. High, untreated cholesterol levels can increase the risk of PAD from 5-fold to 10-fold when compared to subjects with lower cholesterol levels. A high total cholesterol and

142

a low good cholesterol (HDL) can increase the relative risk to develop PAD up to 3.9 times when compared to patients with low total cholesterol and high HDL. Treatment with certain drugs such as **statins** can reduce the incidence of pain during walking in patients with PAD. Statins are also important drugs to reduce **cardiovascular problems** in patients with documented PAD and their use in these patients is warranted.

Obesity and PAD: Is there a relationship?
Obesity is also a significant risk factor to develop plaques in the arteries leading to PAD. In one study, body fat was strongly associated with higher **inflammation markers** and **clotting factors** in the blood stream, both indicate a higher risk to develop PAD and cardiovascular complications. Obesity is part of the **metabolic syndrome**, a diagnosis made when someone has 3 out of the following 5 risk factors: diabetes, obesity, high blood pressure, high **triglycerides** and low good cholesterol. The metabolic syndrome indicates that a person's body is generally resistant to **insulin**. Insulin is a hormone that the pancreas secretes to allow us to use sugar effectively in our body. The prevalence of the metabolic syndrome is 58% in PAD patients, 41% in patients with heart disease, 43% in patients with history of **stroke** and 47% in patients with **abdominal aneurysm**. **Increase in waist fat** is the most important factor that predicts PAD. After controlling for smoking, diabetes, high blood pressure, good cholesterol levels and

triglycerides, an increase in **waist-to-hip ratio** increased independently the risk of PAD by 1.68 times.

Does high blood pressure contribute to PAD?

High blood pressure (**hypertension**) independently increases the risk of PAD by 1.75 times. High blood pressure is also a risk for strokes and heart attacks, and it is of paramount importance to have patients' blood pressure well-controlled. **Exercise**, **limiting salt intake** and **losing weight** are the most important initial steps in lowering blood pressure. However, patients with high blood pressure often require several **blood pressure medications** to treat this problem. Current guidelines suggest a blood pressure below 135/85 mmHg for non-diabetics and a blood pressure below 125/80 for diabetics.

Good nutrition and PAD

PAD is a disease of **plaque build-up** that affects the lower extremity arteries. It is the same process that affects the heart arteries and the arteries of the brain. **Nutritional guidelines** are therefore the same to prevent plaque buildup anywhere in the vascular system. Dietary guidelines that have been widely disseminated apply to patients with PAD. A good diet coupled with exercise allows patients to control their weight and significantly improve many of their cardiovascular risk factors, such as high blood pressure and diabetes. Also, a good diet provides a happier state of mind, a higher energy level and likely more productive life. Poor nutrition has been linked to many chronic disease states that contribute to more disabilities. If you have a specific problem such as hypertension or diabetes or high cholesterol, it is helpful to discuss specific dietary interventions that address your condition. Diets can be tailored to specific disease states to get the most benefit from them. A dietary consultation is generally obtained with a dietitian expert.

What are the general principles for a good diet?

In 2005 the US Government released revised dietary guidelines for Americans. The new *food pyramid* can be found online at: **http://www.mypyramid.gov/downloads/ miniposter.pdf**. This pyramid replaced the old "four basic food groups" that kids grew up with in the 70s. The pyramid continues to promote a variety of food with more emphasis on reducing fat and increasing vitamins and fibers. Disease prevention is an important focus of the new pyramid.

Recommendations per day for a healthy diet for the average adult over the age of 50 include:

- **Grains (at least 3 oz. daily):** Make half of your grains whole grain.1 ounce = about 1 slice bread, about 1 cup of breakfast cereal, or ½ cup cooked rice, pasta or cereal.
- **Vegetables (2-1/2 cups daily):** Eat more dark green veggies and dark leafy greens. Also eat more orange vegetables (like

145

carrots) and more dry beans and peas. If you are on coumadin, you need to consult with your doctor as dark green vegetables contain vitamin K, which can antagonize coumadin function.

- **Fruits (2 cups daily):** Go easy on fruit juice.
- **Milk, yogurt and cheese (3 cups):** Go low-fat or fat-free. 1 cup = 1 cup milk or yogurt, 1 ½ ounces natural cheese or 2 ounces processed cheese.
- **Meat and beans (5-5 ½ oz.):** Chose low-fat or lean meat and poultry. 1 ounce =1 oz. meat, poultry or fish, ¼ cup cooked dry beans, 1 egg, 1 tablespoon peanut butter, ½ oz. nuts or seeds
- Fats, oils and sweets: Use sparingly.

For more information about dietary interventions, calories, weight management and detailed information about fat, carbohydrates, vitamins, minerals and others, please refer to the dietary guidelines 2005 for Americans on the web:
http://www.health.gov/dietaryguidelines/ dga2005/document/

Good nutrition and prevention of disease
Fruits, vegetables, nuts, whole grains, and seeds produce numerous vitamins and phytochemicals are natural substances that allow them to protect themselves against viruses, bacteria and fungi. These substances have been shown to offer prevention against diabetes, high blood pressure, heart disease and cancer. For the PAD patient, these nutrients are important as

they help in the fight against the risk factors of vascular disease:

- Beans, berries, nuts, whole grains and flax seeds that can favorably alter cholesterol to protect the blood vessels
- Cold-water fish such as sardines and salmon contain omega-3 fatty acids that lower the risk for heart attack, high blood pressure and stroke.
- Garlic lowers cholesterol and blood pressure.
- White, green, oolong or black teas (but not herbal teas) may reduce plaque build-up in the arteries. If you are taking coumadin, you should NOT drink green or herbal teas.

Chapter 14

Drugs That Help Patients with Peripheral Arterial Disease
Nicolas W. Shammas, MD, MS

There are few drugs that offer some help to the PAD patients. These can be divided into two major categories: 1) drugs that help in reducing the symptoms of *claudication;* these include cilostazol and statins; and 2) drugs that reduce *cardiovascular events*; these include statins and antiplatelet drugs such as clopidogrel (Plavix) and aspirin. Below is a brief discussion of these drugs or drug classes.

Cilostazol (pletal)
Cilostazol (pletal) is a pharmacologic agent that has been shown to increase walking distance by 54% after 24 weeks of treatment. Cilostazol has been proven to be superior in reducing claudication symptoms than placebo or the commonly prescribed drug *pentoxifylline*, or *Trental*. Cilostazol also reduces the ability of the platelets to clump and cause clots, dilates the blood vessels and improves to a limited extent the cholesterol profile of patients. Cilostazol should not be given in patients with *congestive heart failure* and

should be avoided in patients likely to develop heart failure, such as those with reduced heart function. Cilostazol has been given in some patients before and after an angioplasty to the arteries of the lower legs because it might be helpful in reducing some the **scar tissue** build-up following the procedure.

Statins

Statins are a group of drugs that limit the production of cholesterol from the liver. Statins also have other properties, such as improving the health of the lining of the arteries, reduces plaque build-up and in patients with cardiovascular disease can reduce **stroke**s, **heart attacks** and **claudication** symptoms. Statins have been shown to reduce claudication and increase walking distance by 24% at 6 months and 42% at 1 year. Statins are also essential to reduce cardiovascular events in patients with **atherosclerotic disease** irrespective of **lipid levels**. **Simvastatin** has been shown to significantly increase exercise time until onset of claudication by 24% at 6 months and 42% at 1 year after treatment. Other studies have shown that high-dose, short-term therapy with simvastatin has helped some PAD patients improve their walking performance, symptoms of claudication and the severity of blood reduction to the legs. A low threshold to use statins in PAD patients is warranted.

Antiplatelet drugs

Antiplatelet therapy – **aspirin** or **clopidogrel (Plavix)** or **ticlopidine (Ticlid)** – has not been shown to improve symptoms of claudication but is important to reduce cardiovascular complications associated with the presence of **atherosclerosis** and PAD. A low-dose aspirin (75-150 mg) reduces vascular events by 32% in the high-risk patient including the subset of patients with PAD. "Serious vascular events" including heart attacks, strokes or death were reduced in patients receiving antiplatelet drugs. Clopidogrel (Plavix) was more effective than aspirin in reducing stroke, heart attacks or **vascular death**. Ticlopidine (Ticlid) also has protective effects probably similar to clopidogrel in the high-risk vascular patient but its adverse side effects have limited its use. An infrequent, but serious side effect of Ticlid includes the breakdown of red blood cells (**hemolysis**), and a drop in the number of white blood cells and platelets associated with fever and neurologic changes.

The long-term use (beyond one year) of the clopidogrel-aspirin combination compared to aspirin alone was recently evaluated. Clopidogrel added to aspirin was not significantly more effective than aspirin alone in reducing the rate of heart attack, stroke or death from cardiovascular causes in the stable patients at high risk for cardiovascular events or in patients with established cardiovascular disease. However, many patients stayed on long-term treatment with the combination drugs of aspirin and clopidogrel if their doctors felt they are very high risk for recurrent cardiovascular events.

Is there any role for vitamins to treat the PAD patient?

Currently there is no data to support that taking **vitamins** is helpful in treating patients with PAD or other cardiovascular diseases. Vitamin E and Vitamin C have been shown in large studies to have no impact on improving the outcome of patients with cardiovascular disease or at risk of developing cardiovascular disease. In fact, Vitamin E does negatively interfere with the effectiveness of statins and is best avoided in these patients. **Folic acid** (or **folate**) also showed to have no impact on the prognosis of high risk of cardiovascular patients. At this time, we do not recommend vitamins for patients with PAD as there is no data to support their use.

How about fish oil and the PAD patient?

Fish oil has not been tested specifically in patients with PAD but has been evaluated in patients at increased risk of cardiovascular events and PAD falls into this category. Fish oil at 1000 mg per day can improve a patient's **cholesterol profile** by lowering the **bad cholesterol** (**LDL**) and improving the **good cholesterol** (**HDL**). Also, it has been shown to reduce cardiovascular death in high-risk cardiac patients. Fish oil is therefore a good adjunctive treatment to well-established medications such as the statins.

Although we note from this chapter that the list of medications that can be helpful to the PAD patient is limited, nonetheless these medications are important and treatment with these

152

medications can improve a patient's symptoms and outcome.

Chapter 15

A Collaborative Team Approach in the Fight Against PAD
Penny Stoakes, RN, BS, CCRC
Desyree Weakley, RN, CRC

Primary Prevention of Peripheral Arterial Disease in Adults
A growing body of evidence supports the promise of primary prevention of high blood cholesterol. Primary prevention of **high blood cholesterol** (**hyperlipidemia/dyslipidemia**) should be an important aspect of the societal approach to the promotion of good cardiovascular health.

In this chapter, **cardiovascular health** encompasses an array of terms, including **peripheral artery disease**, **coronary artery disease**, **atherosclerosis**, **coronary heart disease**, **cerebrovascular disease**, and **carotid artery disease**.

What are lipids? How are they related to high blood cholesterol?
The word "**lipid**" comes from the Greek "lipos," which means "fat." Lipids are organic compounds (including **fats**, **oils**, **waxes**, **sterols**, or

glycerides) that are insoluble in water but soluble in organic solvents. Research indicates a direct relationship between **cholesterol triglyceride levels** and the development of **coronary artery disease** (**CAD**), or **plugged arteries**.

What is case management?
Case management provides systematic evaluation and implementation of medical treatments with regular follow-up of those at risk for a cardiac or vascular event. Evidence suggests that **case management** results in an increase in short-term compliance and a reduction in both emergency room visits and hospitalizations.

Why is case management helpful to people with high blood cholesterol?
Patients perceive that they need **individualized education** and **counseling**, as well as skills to help them set goals and resolve difficulties with **lifestyle changes**. They respond well to a planned approach to accessing the medical care system appropriately. The ability to help them identify and sort out symptoms supports their overall health. Finally, **case management systems** also help patients and family members identify appropriate community resources.

Effectiveness of a **collaborative approach to case management** has been well-documented during the last two decades, both in the United States and globally. Case management has been shown to be an effective method to the

156

management of high blood cholesterol and multiple risk factors in a number of populations. In addition, this approach to managing high-risk populations has shown improved outcomes as evidenced by a reduction in **_morbidity and mortality rates_**.

Medical therapies are complex and require patient education, systematic medical follow-up, and ongoing management. A collaborative approach among nursing, nutrition, and medicine will provide improved patient compliance, greater ability to reach lipid goals, and greater safety. A major benefit of a collaborative approach to medical therapies is the improved access that patients generally have when faced with questions and/or concerns such as those regarding side effects. Support and "patient connection" can be provided through mail, telephone, fax, and the Internet. These methods can save costs by reducing emergency department visits, unnecessary physician's office visits, and poor patient compliance.

Coronary Heart Disease Prevention in Adults: A Collaborative Approach

- Administered by nurses, health educators, and/or other healthcare providers
- Adherence to recommendations of national healthcare organizations (i.e., American Heart Association [AHA], American College of Cardiology [ACC], National Institutes of Health [NIH])
- Open and regular communication with clinical experts and the medical community

- Responsibility for the organization and collection of data for individual and clinical populations

Success depends on attention to multiple tasks:
- Titration of medications
- Management of side effects
- Use of combination therapies
- Use of lower-cost medications
- Behavioral interventions for lifestyle modification

What role can nutrition play in the management of lipids?

The role of the nutritionist cannot be understated. Effective **nutrition education** and support can improve **blood lipids** and **body weight** through the intake of **heart-healthy foods** and **caloric restriction**, improve physical activity levels; reduce insulin resistance; improve the health of people with Type 2 diabetes mellitus who control their glucose; and decrease the development of Type 2 diabetes. The inclusion of nutrition is key to a collaborative approach.

What are the American Heart Association Recommendations for Achieving Desirable Blood Lipid Profile and Especially LDL-C?
- Limit foods high in saturated fats
- Replace saturated fats with lower-fat foods
- Increase type of foods with unsaturated fat
- Carefully monitor intake of food high in

158

cholesterol
- Severely limit foods containing trans fatty acids
- Increase foods rich in viscous fiber
- Increase foods containing stanol/sterol esters (special margarines, fortified orange juice, special cocoa/chocolate bars)

What is the impact of Physical Activity on Blood Lipids and Lipoproteins?

Physical activity beneficially influences most of the risk factors for **atherosclerosis**. The impact of regular exercise on **plasma lipids** and **lipoproteins** has been clearly defined with regard to the interactions among lipids, lipoproteins, **apolipoproteins** (**apo**), **lipoprotein enzymes**, and the influence of various factors such as **aging**, **body fat distribution**, **dietary composition**, and **cigarette smoking** status.

As with nutrition, the importance of **physical activity** cannot be underestimated.

A collaborative approach to the care of adults with coronary risk factors through the use of non-physician healthcare providers such as **nutritionists**, **nurses**, and **exercise physiologists** can help improve patients' success in the adoption of regular physical activity. **Cardiac rehabilitation programs** can offer assistance to healthcare providers with exercise education and supervision when indicated – another method of enhancing a collaborative approach to risk reduction.

Significant changes can be seen in lipid and lipoprotein/lipid concentrations after just a single exercise session. However, to maintain these beneficial changes, exercise must be performed regularly.

Therefore, physical activity and exercise training are strongly encouraged, 5 to 7 days a week, for at least 30 minutes per day, and 60 minutes per day for people who need to achieve weight loss. If this is done with an appropriate emphasis on nutrition and adherence to other recommendations by providers, then body fat likely will be reduced, and the need for medication therapy may be less in some people.

Developing a system for collaborating with healthcare providers who have expertise in behavior change, exercise science for adults, and nutrition will support the important role of regular physical activity in lipid management and overall risk reduction.

What is drug therapy, and how is it helpful in managing high blood cholesterol?
Medical therapies (i.e., medications prescribed by doctors) for high blood cholesterol are key for people at high risk for the disease and for people with known atherosclerosis. A collaborative approach to medical therapies, often prescribed for a lifetime, has been shown to improve patient compliance and quality of life. Millions of Americans remain at risk from high blood cholesterol, in spite of safe and effective treatments. Implementing a collaborative

160

approach through the inclusion of nutritionists and nurses is the key to long-term maintenance and safety of medical therapies.

Although effective drugs now exist to improve lipid profiles, no single drug is most appropriate under all circumstances. The appropriate treatment of the most common lipid abnormalities includes the use of the following classes of drugs: **statins**, **resins**, **niacin**, and **fibrates**, as well as **fish oil**, either singly or in combination.

When is it appropriate to consider the use of supplements in the management of abnormal blood lipids?

There are no available, well-tested **supplements** that achieve the magnitude of lipid lowering that is observed with traditional pharmaceutical therapies. With the exception of **plant stanols** and **omega-3 fatty acids**, most supplements have demonstrated only a small beneficial effect on blood lipids. Thus, current data suggest a limit role for supplements in the treatment of abnormal blood lipids. Patient education regarding the benefits and risks of **vitamins** and **supplements** is an integral and important component in the treatment of dyslipidemia. Nutritionists are well-positioned to provide information about supplements – an additional key reason for collaboration.

What is adherence and why is it important for patients?

"*Adherence*" is a medical term referring to the

patient "following" or "sticking to" the directives of the health care professional.

In no other arena is collaboration more important than when considering adherence. Behavioral science, social science, psychology, and medicine meet at this crossroads. Through collaborative efforts, adherence to important lifesaving interventions can be positively influenced.

Treatment of high blood cholesterol may include a special eating plan, weight reduction, smoking cessation, regular exercise, and/or lipid-lowering medications. Although this therapeutic plan may represent the optimal treatment approach, it also highlights the challenges facing patients who are attempting to incorporate these changes into their lives.

As with many patient-related factors, these situations call for an open dialogue between patient and provider that encourages the patient to examine the risks and benefits of the treatment with the guidance of the healthcare professional. The ability to maintain open communication with the patient will permit a discussion of many factors that may influence a patient's compliance and will go far in enhancing patient adherence.

How does high blood cholesterol affect coronary artery disease (CAD), cerebrovascular disease (stroke), and peripheral arterial disease (PAD)?

High cholesterol (dyslipidemia) has been determined to be one of the causative factors in coronary artery disease (CAD), cerebrovascular disease (stroke), and peripheral arterial disease. It is clear that a collaborative approach to administering lifestyle changes in conjunction with a systematic approach to the use of effective lipid-lowering medications will maximize the likelihood that patients will attain well-accepted risk factor goals and will minimize the likelihood of preventable coronary events. Extensive clinical trial data document the effects of pharmacological lipid-lowering therapy on clinical outcomes in patients with these three conditions.

In conclusion . . . .

Collaboration within the healthcare community is an ongoing and fluent process. Patients may first be diagnosed with **PAD** by their ***primary doctor*** and then referred to a ***podiatrist***, ***wound clinic***, or even an ***endovascular cardiologist*** or ***vascular surgeon***. If a patient is already established within a cardiology practice, then a diagnosis may originate from that specialist. Multiple factors affect referrals, including ***physician awareness of specialists and treatment options***, ***patient preference***, and ***insurance coverage***. ***Open communication***, ***continuous networking***, and ***ongoing education*** are essential to promote not only healthy relationships among various practices (e.g., ***family practice doctors***, ***cardiologists***, ***podiatrists***, ***surgeons***) and other

interdisciplinary teams (e.g., **dietitians,** *nurses,* **exercise physiologists**), but also updating knowledge of how the different providers are treating their patient populations and utilizing new therapies and strategies.

Chapter 16

The Research to Fight PAD: How You Can Help
Lori Christensen, RN
Denise Coiner, MS, RTR

What is a clinical trial?
A *clinical trial* is a scientific study in humans to evaluate the effects of new medications or devices. Each trial has specific goals or objectives that need to be met in order to get accurate results. These studies are the basis for companies to develop new products that could be beneficial to many people.

What are the phases of clinical research?
Phase I: Investigational drug is given to humans for the first time. This phase only enrolls a small number of healthy subjects to determine the safety of the drug, study how it is absorbed and eliminated in the body, and find the best dose to be tested in a larger number of patients.

Phase II: These subjects have the target disease in which the investigational drug or device is being tested. This phase is also testing for efficacy but also assesses safety.

Phase III: This phase has a large population of

subjects. The purpose of this phase is to determine long-term safety and effectiveness in a larger number of subjects before releasing the investigational drug or device to the market.

Each phase is very important and critical in evaluating the safety of the drug or device.

Is it safe to participate in clinical research? Participating in research is optional, and you should never feel obligated to participate. There are special measures that are taken to ensure your safety throughout the trial, including visits with clinical research nurses and/or a nurse practitioner or physician periodically throughout the clinical trial duration. Physical exams generally are done at every visit, providing the opportunity to discuss any issues you might be having that need further evaluation. Other testing could also be done at your study visits and could include blood work and EKGs. As with any medication or device, there can be side effects. These are outlined in the ***informed consent form***, which provides information about the clinical trial and outlines your rights as a research subject. In any clinical trial, it is important to monitor your health, and any changes need to be reported to the study staff.

Is my privacy protected when I get involved in research? Yes. The federal government has implemented **HIPPA** (***Health Insurance Portability and Accountability Act***) to protect your rights to control access to and disclosure of your private and confidential information. If you choose to participate in a research study, you will be asked to sign a specific authorization for release of any of your health information for research purposes only. You will also be asked to sign an informed consent prior to participating in the study.

What is the research coordinator's role in the research trial?
The *clinical research coordinator* works under the direction of the *principal investigator*, the PI, who is the physician who oversees the trial. There are many roles a research coordinator handles during the course of a trial. These include assisting in evaluating new studies, preparing the site for conducting the study, reviewing patients' symptoms to see if they qualify for studies, participating in the informed consent process and managing study conduct throughout the study. The clinical research coordinator will collect all of your information at each study visit and will be the primary person you see throughout the duration of the clinical trial.

Why is getting involved in clinical research so important?
The healthcare field is always evolving, with new *technology* being developed and implemented all of the time. This is also true for new medications or new devices from which patients can benefit. In order to see if such things are beneficial, they have to go through the clinical research trials to determine their efficacy

and safety in patients. Although you may not benefit directly from the experimental device or medication at the time of the study, your participation has a great impact on healthcare. You are part of the information that is generated from the clinical research trial to obtain the end results that could lead to the approval of such new medications or devices.

What is the impact of clinical research on the current treatment of the PAD patients?
All clinical research trials have a great impact on treatment. There are many different research trials that involve patients with PAD (peripheral artery disease). These trials focus on different *blood vessels* in the legs that have blockages and are testing different ways to treat these blood vessels. The impact with these research trials can be very beneficial in answering specific questions for the treatment of PAD. The main impact of research on PAD patients is to improve the quality and prolong the life of these patients. Various drugs also are being tested to also reduce the incidence of *strokes* and *heart attacks* in these patients. In addition, various devices have been developed to unplug *blockages* in the blood vessels in the lower legs to improve the ability of a patient to *walk* and *exercise*.

What are some of the current areas of research in PAD?
There are *device and drug trials* that currently are being done to evaluate new areas of treatment for patients with PAD. Depending on

168

the degree and severity of your PAD, you might qualify for one of these trials. There are studies being conducted for patients that have PAD in certain blood vessels in their legs or for patients that have non-healing ulcers present.

Some treatments include:

Balloon angioplasty: Insertion of an angioplasty balloon to dilate the artery.

Stenting: A wire mesh tube is inserted in the artery and expanded with a balloon to keep the artery open.

Atherectomy: A device that shaves the inside wall of the artery and removes the plaque that has formed there.

Rotoblating: A device that spins at a high rate of speed and pulverizes the plaque inside the artery wall.

Aspiration and infusion catheters: Treatments with catheters that infuse a clot-busting drug and remove the clot through the catheter.

Distal Embolic Protection Devices: A small basket that is distal to the treatment that is being performed that catches any particles that might slough off from the treatment and prevents the particles from occluding distal vessels.

Laser Atherectomy: A catheter that uses light waves to ablate plaque in the blood vessel.

Angiogenesis: Research with drugs that help promote the development of new blood vessels in patients with end-stage non-treatable disease at risk of losing their legs.

Antirestenosis studies: Trials designed to find drugs and devices that prevent the recurrence of blockage after the initial treatment.

An invitation to participate in clinical research: Be part of the history of science!
Being part of a clinical research trial can be very rewarding. The results of the research trials can definitely make a difference in treatments we see in the future for certain diseases. Knowing that you were part of this experience that can change the face of medicine can be quite rewarding. Knowing that you have helped future generations to live a better lifestyle and knowing that just maybe it would be your own children or grandchildren that would benefit makes participating in research a worthwhile effort.

Chapter 17

Saving Legs and Lives: Together We Can Do It
Nicolas W. Shammas, MD, MS

If you are reading this book, you are already on the right track to taking care of yourself. It all starts with educating yourself about the symptoms and signs of PAD, its risk factors, how to modify your risk and when to report to your doctor. We are hoping that we have provided you with some basic information to help you reach these goals. The field of PAD is changing rapidly, and keeping yourself educated about your disease is important. The following are some useful web pages that can help you stay up-to-date on PAD:

* http://www.mayoclinic.com/health/peripheral-arterial-disease/DS00537
* http://www.nlm.nih.gov/medlineplus/peripheralarterialdisease.html
* http://www.hearthub.org/hc-peripheral.htm
* http://www.hearthub.org/hc-stroke.htm
* http://www.nhlbi.nih.gov/health/public/heart/pad/index.html
* http://www.sirweb.org/patients/peripheral-arterial-disease/

Furthermore, attending local seminars by healthcare professionals and community health fairs can also provide you with some important tips about diet and weight-loss programs and might allow you access to some screening tests such as blood pressure measurements, screening for PAD, cholesterol and blood sugar testing.

It is also very important for patients to be compliant with their doctor's recommendations. Remember that patients infrequently die of PAD itself but mostly of associated complications related to heart disease and strokes. It is therefore important to ensure that all your cardiac risk factors are under control, including your blood pressure, diabetes, cholesterol, weight, diet and exercise. Quitting smoking is also probably one of the most important step you can take to protect your heart, brain, legs and life. Taking your medications faithfully, particularly your cholesterol drugs and your blood thinners (aspirin and/or clopidogrel), will significantly reduce your chance of cardiovascular problems. Routine exercise and diet are of paramount importance. Patients should not feel that they can lead a sedentary life and eat whatever they like because their cholesterol or blood pressure levels are controlled with medications. One needs to remember that some of the best treatment for PAD is exercise and quitting smoking that prolongs substantially a person's ability to walk and lead a better quality of life.

Patients with advanced PAD and non-healing leg wounds need to have an aggressive evaluation for PAD before an amputation is performed. It is important that patients are aware that amputations in the US are quite often performed without screening for PAD or an attempt to treat the impaired blood supply to the leg. Current treatment technologies can lead to a successful restoration of blood supply to the affected leg in over 90% of patients and data suggest that saving a leg in these patients is achievable in over 90% of the time.

In summary, leading a healthy lifestyle, getting education about PAD and the drugs that you take and being compliant with your doctor's visit and recommendations will certainly protect you from PAD and its complications, prolong your life and improve its quality. Saving legs and life . . . together we can do it!